Father

OF THE

Blind

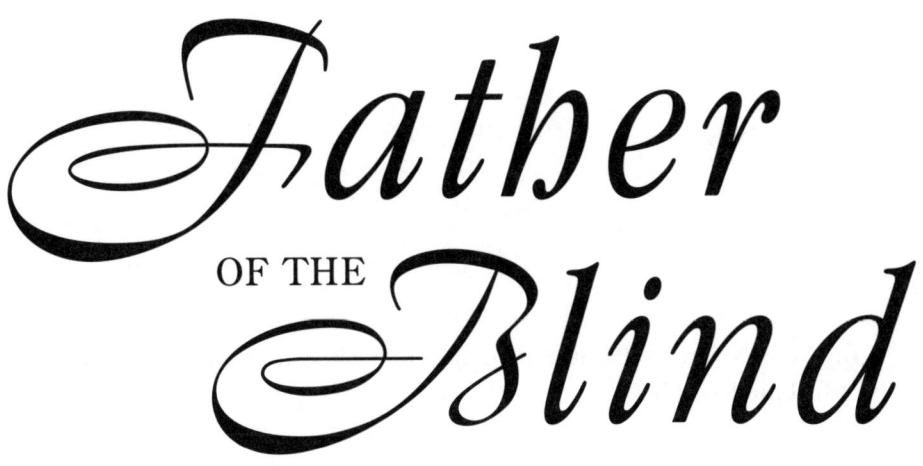

Father

OF THE Blind

A PORTRAIT OF SIR ARTHUR PEARSON

ANDREW NORMAN

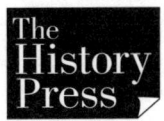

The History Press

Dedication

To my beloved late grandfather, St Dunstaner Thomas Waldin, formerly of the 8th Rifle Brigade.

Jacket Illustration: Arthur Pearson. Photo: St Dunstan's.

First published 2009

The History Press
The Mill, Brimscombe Port
Stroud, Gloucestershire, GL5 2QG
www.thehistorypress.co.uk

British Library Cataloguing in Publication Data.
A catalogue record for this book is available from the British Library.

ISBN 978 0 7524 5182 4

Typesetting and origination by The History Press
Printed in Great Britain

Contents

Foreword

This well-researched and highly readable book describes the life and work of my late grandfather Sir Arthur Pearson, founder of the *Daily Express* newspaper.

When, in middle-life, Sir Arthur became blind, he used his business acumen, expertise, and connections to help others in a similar predicament. He infected everyone with his enthusiasm and determination to achieve 'Victory over Blindness'.

Sir Arthur is remembered for his many acts of charity, including the creation of the Fresh Air Fund for children, However, he is chiefly remembered as the founder of St Dunstan's, which gave hope and purpose to the blinded British and Allied soldiers of World War I.

Sally Hardy
(granddaughter of Sir Arthur Pearson)

Acknowledgements

I am grateful to the following: Canadian National Institute for the Blind; National Federation of the Blind, USA; Helen Keller International; Royal New Zealand Foundation of the Blind; South African National Council for the Blind; Veterans Affairs, Canada; Vision Australia.

Thanks to the British Medical Association; Brotherton Library, Leeds; City of Westminster Archives Centre; Poole Central Library; Imperial War Museum; IPC London; Islington and Camden Cemetery Services; Moorfields Eye Hospital and Institute of Ophthalmology; National Army Museum; Pearson's Holiday Fund; Royal College of Anaesthetists; Royal College of Ophthalmologists; Royal College of Physicians of England; Royal College of Surgeons of England; Royal Green Jackets' Museum, Winchester; Somerset County Museums Service; The Scout Association; Winchester College Archives.

The following individuals have most helpful: Peter Adams; John B. Atkins; Alan Baker; D. J. Bignell; Colonel Ian Causland; Gabriel Dragffy; Marian Gotto; Major K. Gray; Judith Haswell; Penny Hatfield; His Honour Judge Nicholas Huskinson; Charlie Jacoby; Peter Kazmierczak; Richard Keeler; Louise King; Jane Lindstrand-Gotto; Marian Gotto; Alastair Massie; Mark Quinlan; Bryan K. H. Rogers; Theo V. Thomas; Lynda Unchern.

Also a thank you to members of my family, Jean Norman, Jane Savery, Peter, David and Howard Waldin for their kindness in loaning photographs, and for sharing their memories with me.

I am especially grateful to Sir Arthur Pearson's granddaughter Sally Hardy, and to my beloved wife Rachel for all their help and encouragement.

The views expressed in this book are solely those of the author, and have not been endorsed or authorised by St Dunstan's.

Author's Note

It is Sunday, 21 July 1947. I am 4 years old and sitting outside in a deckchair in the garden of a house in Winchester, Hampshire. Seeking to amuse me, my maternal grandfather begins to pull the deckchair across the grass. As he is blind, he fails to notice my expression change but my laughter turns to screams as the index finger of my left hand had become jammed in the hinge. Hearing the commotion, Thomas's mother-in-law – my great grandmother Jane Benwell – comes rushing out of the house and before I know it, she is pouring iodine from a blue bottle, over the wound. She then replaces the flap of skin that is hanging off the finger and applies a bandage. She scolds Thomas severely; whereupon he also begins to weep. To see him so upset makes me cry even more. Only now is the family doctor summoned. Dr Bliss tells Mrs Benwell that she has done exactly the right thing, and presents her with a bill for £1.10s.

I knew that my grandfather had been blinded during the First World War. I was also aware that he wore an enamelled badge, bearing the words 'St Dunstan's' with the motif of a flaming torch. Also, that the family had named the house where they lived 'St Dunstan's'. It was more than 50 years, however, before I learnt the full story of what he had experienced; of the circumstances of his blinding and of how a wonderful man named Cyril Arthur Pearson had come to his aid when he was in the depths of despair.

Preface

The year might be any one between 1915 and 1920; the place, a workshop in the grounds of a London mansion. From this workshop emanates the deafening sound of men, 50 or so in number, hammering nails into hobnail boots. Competing with this cacophony is the sound of the men's voices. They are singing – confident songs such as 'It's a Long Way to Tipperary,' or songs of tenderness and nostalgia, like 'There's a Long, Long Trail a Winding'. Their 'Cobblers' Chorus' echoes the pleasure they feel in what they are doing. But how can this be? How *can* they be happy, when less than a year previously, these very same men were experiencing the hell of the battlefield: being shelled, bombed, mined, shot at, gassed and finally, in their case, blinded? The change in their attitude and demeanour was nothing short of miraculous, and who had brought about this apparent miracle? A man called Arthur Pearson whom the men called the 'Chief'.

In 1915, the second year of the First World War, Pearson founded St Dunstan's, a hostel for the care and rehabilitation of soldiers and sailors who had been blinded in the conflict. This was a time when the Western Front, that great, insentient and seemingly insatiable killing machine (and also other theatres of war such as Gallipoli, the Dardanelles and the Persian Gulf) was currently gobbling men up on an unimaginable scale, before regurgitating them bleeding, broken, and sometimes, sightless.

The challenge faced by Pearson was an enormous one. The servicemen he wished to help were, in the main, proud men from Britain and the British Empire, who had gone to war with every expectation of a quick success. Instead, they had found themselves hopelessly bogged down in theatres such as the Armageddon-like Western Front. Included in their number were the limbless, the maimed, the shell-shocked, the paralysed and the deaf. In addition to these depredations, all of them, mostly young men in the prime of their lives, were also blind.

One might imagine that their thoughts were: 'Why am I still here, when most of my comrades are dead?' 'Will my wife/mother/girlfriend still love me when they see me like this?' 'How will I manage to feed and dress myself and find my way around?' 'How can I afford to live?' 'Where will I find friends, such as those I knew in the army?' Those men from distant places – Australia, New Zealand, Canada, Rhodesia and South Africa – who had no hope of receiving a visit from their relatives, would have felt particularly bereft. Given all these seemingly insurmountable problems and the fact that Pearson was not trained in psychology, how did he possibly hope to succeed? And yet he did succeed, and one of the reasons for his success was the fact that he too was blind.

Although it is for the founding of St Dunstan's that Pearson is chiefly remembered, there were many other fascinating aspects to his life. He created a famous newspaper, the *Daily Express*; he enabled Baden-Powell to launch the Boy Scout Movement; he financed an expedition to find the giant sloth of South America – hitherto believed to be extinct. Equally intriguing is Pearson's own struggle. How was this talented and energetic man to cope with eyesight which had gradually deteriorated since schooldays, and which he finally lost completely at the age of 48? His interest in the occult – about he which wrote several books – is surely a reflection of his compelling desire to find his way, and foretell what the future held for him. To all outward appearances he was an extrovert who numbered amongst his friends HM Queen Alexandra, Helen Adams Keller, Robert Baden-Powell, and Conservative politician Joseph Chamberlain. Inwardly, evidence is put forward that he was riddled with insecurity, which, given the circumstances in which he found himself, was quite understandable. Nonetheless, he was able to achieve, to use his favourite phrase, 'Victory over Blindness'. This is his story.

1

Arthur Pearson: Early Life

Cyril Arthur Pearson was born on 24 February 1866 at Wookey in Somerset, where his father, the Reverend Arthur Cyril Pearson, was curate at the Church of St Matthew. His mother was Philippa Massingberd Pearson (née Maxwell-Lyte, whose grandfather, the Reverend Henry Francis Lyte, wrote the words to one of the most moving hymns in the English language – 'Abide with Me'.) Pearson had three younger sisters – Mabel, Marion and Olive.

From 1876, Pearson attended Eagle House Preparatory School in Wimbledon where he showed potential at cricket, as a promising bowler. In 1877, the Reverend A.C. Pearson became Rector of Drayton Parslow in Buckinghamshire.

Following in the footsteps of his father, Pearson commenced as a pupil at Winchester College public school in Hampshire, southern England, entering that establishment in January 1880 as a Commoner in 'D' House. Given the nickname 'Pigeon', he proved to be both popular and sociable. Pearson was 'always up to some merry prank or other, was famous for telling the funniest stories night after night' and he (and his father) were 'wonderful hands at riddles, puzzles, chess problems, acrostics, and tricks of all kinds'.[1] In fact, the Reverend Pearson would go on to have books published on such subjects, including *One Hundred Chess Problems* (1878),

The Twentieth Century Standard Puzzle Book, and *The Twentieth Century Standard Problem Book* (both 1907; the latter being devoted to the solving of mathematical problems – or 'recreational mathematics'). Not to be outdone, his wife Philippa published *The Acrostic Dictionary* (1901). At the end of his first term, Pearson was awarded prize money – for the purchase of books – after coming top of his class.

Pearson threw himself enthusiastically into sport, he played cricket for his house (his father before him had played for the School's 1st XI) and gained a reputation for being 'a most tricky bowler amongst the Juniors'.[2] On the annual athletics day in 1881, he competed in an event listed as the 'Wide [long] Jump – For all under 5ft 4in and 16 years';

> This [event] was easily won by Pearson, with an extremely fine jump, which he accomplished after several attempts, in the greater number of which he fell backwards and lost his jump. Grant and Hardy were the next best, but considerably behind Pearson.

In the following year, 1882, he competed in the hurdles, 100 yards, and 200 yards flat races, and wide jump.[3] Pearson also enjoyed hockey and lawn tennis. In fact, outwardly, all appeared to be well with him, both at work and play. However, in reality this was far from the case, for as Gerald Fiennes, one of his contemporaries said of him brutally, but nonetheless truthfully: 'he was too blind to play games well'.[4] Alas, matters could only get worse.

Pearson's time at Winchester College was to be cut short. In early 1882, when he was sixteen and had been at the school for only two years, he was prematurely withdrawn as his father could no longer afford to pay the fees. He was now 'thrown on the world, penniless, with no prospect before him'.[5]

Despite the fact that at Winchester College Pearson had developed problems with his eyesight, this did not prevent him from sending articles which he had written to a weekly magazine called *Tit-Bits*. Founded by Sir George Newnes in Manchester in 1881, *Tit-Bits* was so successful that its editorial office was moved to London.

On 31 May 1884, while Pearson was waiting (perhaps not with bated breath) to hear about a promised vacancy at a City of London bank, he noticed an advertisement on *Tit-Bits'* front page. 'AN EXTRAORDINARY PRIZE' was offered, namely:

A SITUATION
in the Offices of *Tit-Bits*,
at a Salary of £100 per annum.

To win the prize it was necessary to answer, correctly, questions on general knowledge, ten of which would appear in each of the next thirteen editions of the magazine.

Pearson realised that if he was to have a chance of winning, he would have to travel 30 miles to the town of Bedford where he could discover the answers in the town's library. This he did, no less than three times per week, on a high-wheeled bicycle (one in which the front wheel is larger than the rear wheel) which he had recently learned to ride. On 26 September 1884 the result was announced. Out of 3,000 competitors, Pearson had won with 86 correct answers out of a possible 130. That same month, he took lodgings in Wimbledon and commenced work for George Newnes at his publishing house in London, in fact on a salary of £350 per annum.

At *Tit-Bits*, Pearson was a great success. Before long, Newnes described him as his 'right-hand man' and he was awarded his own private secretary Ernest Kessell, who had only recently left school. In his spare time, Pearson displayed the caring nature which would become his hallmark: 'He would hire an omnibus, into which he would personally pack a company of poor London children, and send them up for a blow on Hampstead Heath. It was part of his nature to love and cheer little children.'[6]

Six months after Pearson joined *Tit-Bits*, its manager suddenly resigned, and Pearson applied for his position. He was refused. Three months later, he applied again but Newnes was hesitant. However, when another three months had passed, Pearson's wish was granted.

The energetic Pearson continued with writing articles, choosing subjects as varied as 'Fireplaces', 'Echoes', 'Royal Authors', 'Steeplejacks' Work', 'Gout', 'Suspended Animation' and 'Duelling'. His aim was both to entertain and to inform. For example, in his article 'Rats', which was published by *The Cornhill Magazine*,[7] he wrote: 'The best course to take, when the extermination of a colony of rats becomes a necessity, is to make them help to destroy one another in the following manner.'

He went on to describe how the rats could be enticed with 'a dainty meal of bacon-rind and other scraps,' to gain their confidence. Once this had been achieved, the piece of brown paper on which they were accustomed to stand for their meal, could be cut in such a way that next time, they would be precipitated into a tub of cold water below. The creature would then take refuge on a specially positioned island, from where his alarm calls would be heard by other rats who would thereby be lured into the same trap. The plan, said Pearson, had been tried in a City warehouse, where 'more than three thousand rats were destroyed in a single night'.

Pearson went to great lengths to get his works published. His friend and biographer Sidney Dark said, 'there can hardly have been a newspaper or periodical editor in London whom he did not bombard'.[8] A measure of his success is indicated by Pearson's own records, which show that in 1889, between 1 January and 30 June, no less than 58 out of 84 articles written by him were accepted and published; from which he earned the sum of £44.

In December 1887, when Pearson was aged only 21, he married Isabel Sarah, who, like himself, was the offspring of a clergyman, the Reverend John Bennett of Maddington, Wiltshire. She bore him three daughters, Isla Marion, Muriel and Nora.

In 1889, W. T. Stead, editor of the *Pall Mall Gazette*, founded a monthly journal in partnership with Newnes, the *Review of Reviews*, the name of which is self-explanatory. Within a month Newnes had published the first copy and as Business Manager, Pearson was dispatched to the USA to arrange for it to be sold there.

In view of this, Pearson believed that he deserved a rise in salary. Newnes refused. Pearson, who had worked for the company for almost six years, now decided to leave, as did his secretary Ernest Kessell, together with editor Peter Keary.

2

Pearson's Weekly:
Pearson's Magazine

With the help of his two former colleagues from Newnes – Ernest Kessell and Peter Keary – Pearson created his own company, C. Arthur Pearson Ltd. Within three weeks, with finance provided by Stephen Mills, the new company published the first number of the periodical journal *Pearson's Weekly*, which appeared on 26 July 1890. Writing years later of his father, Pearson's son Sir Neville declared:

> He was a man of immense energy. When he first started in business on his own, for the first week in his office, the only sleep he took was on the office table. He literally worked day and night.[1]

The first issue of *Pearson's Weekly* sold 250,000. In that same year Pearson moved from Wimbledon Common to 'The Bungalow', Shere, Surrey. He would go on to move several more times to other properties in Surrey – 'Round Down', Gomshall (1891); 'Cattershall Manor', Godalming (1895), and 'Broadwater', Godalming (1896).

Pearson is described as having:

> A thick crop of wiry black hair, gold pince-nez glasses, and a small dark moustache. He was totally indifferent to dress, and usually wore, at his office,

a Norfolk jacket and a pique four-in-hand tie with a gold pin. He would not always dress for dinner if he could escape the necessity. If he smoked at all, it was very seldom. Experiments and diets interested him. For long periods he would drink nothing but water; eat only fruit for breakfast, and again in the afternoon, when others were taking tea.[2]

The motto of *Pearson's Weekly* was 'To Interest, to Elevate, to Amuse'. The newspaper was unique in that unlike all similar publications, it carried no advertisements on its front page. At that time, Britain was engaged in a war in South Africa and it was not difficult to fill its pages with news.

Pearson was determined that in its content, quality of debate and presentation, *Pearson's Weekly* would be a cut above other newspapers. There would be factual and informative articles on topics such as 'Domestic Lighting', and on topical questions of the day, such as 'Does Education Diminish Crime?'; fictional stories; a letter page where its readers could express their views; and competitions for prizes. It was no coincidence, bearing in mind that both Pearson's and his wife Isobel's fathers were clergymen and that many in the lower echelons of this profession were obliged to live lives of frugality, that the competition held in the first edition of *Pearson's Weekly* was designed for clergymen, with annuities given as prizes.

Mindful of the fact that his eyesight was continuing to fail, the 24-year-old Pearson produced an article for this very first *Pearson's Weekly* entitled 'Curiosities of Blindness':

Appalling as the deprivation of sight may be, it is not without some remarkable compensations. Other faculties, both of intellect and of sense, often seem to gain by it … Profound thinkers practically admit that vision interferes somewhat with deep cogitation … Men of genius have sometimes thrown off some of the worst disabilities of blindness. Genius ever devises ways and means of its own. It has a thousand little contrivances unknown to the ordinary student, who is content enough to travel along the beaten road which others have fashioned for him.

Pearson then goes on to give, as examples, Nicholas Saunderson, the blind mathematician who became a friend of Sir Isaac Newton and was elected Professor of Mathematics at Cambridge University; John Metcalf, the blind engineer who, 'constructed roads through the wilds of Derbyshire', and Thomas Blacklock, the blind poet and musician who could speak four languages.

Demonstrating his caring and philanthropic nature, within eighteen months of the publication of the first *Pearson's Weekly*, Pearson had collected sufficient money from his readers to be able to provide a Christmas dinner for many hundreds of deprived children from London's East End.

He resorted to many ingenious ploys in order to keep his readership interested. For example, the first 'happy father' who informed *Pearson's Weekly* that his wife had produced twins, was eligible for the prize of £10, which was awarded weekly for four weeks – provided, of course, that the event was confirmed by a birth certificate. From here Pearson proceeded to anticipate the modern phenomenon of newspaper dating, when his single young men and women readers were invited to send in a photograph with a reference. The editor then chose a 'lucky young woman', who was given the choice of ten male applicants, similarly selected, to be her husband. She would also receive £100 a year for life, together with the expenses of her wedding and honeymoon.

Other periodicals followed in the wake of *Pearson's Weekly*: *Home Notes*; *The Royal Magazine*; *The Smallholder*; *The Scout* (about which more will be said shortly); *Peg's Paper*, and *Peg's Companion*.

1896 saw the appearance of the pro-socialist *Pearson's Magazine*, which published articles and short stories by such authors as H. G. Wells, George Bernard Shaw, Maxim Gorky, Upton Sinclair and H. Rider Haggard. Like *Pearson's Weekly*, it also contained articles on science, sport, travel, and invention. In 1899, *Pearson's Magazine* was first published in the USA.

Despite all Pearson's efforts, *Pearson's Weekly* ran into financial difficulties, and Sir William Ingram, the proprietor of the *Illustrated London News*, agreed to take a 49% stake in the company, leaving Pearson with a 51% controlling stake. Pearson, however, retained full ownership of *Pearson's Magazine*.

3

Pearson's Fresh
Air Fund

In the summer of 1892, Pearson launched his Fresh Air Fund, and became its President. In so doing, he was no doubt aware that he was emulating the Reverend Willard Parsons of Sherman, Pennsylvania, USA, who in 1877 had preceded him by founding the American version of this organisation.

In 1949, almost six decades after the event, Pearson's son Sir Neville (by his second wife Ethel Fraser) described how this organisation, something which his mother, 'had been deeply interested in,' had come into being. The fund, he said, was established

> … to enable many thousands of unfortunate children to enjoy the fresh, country air for even a day, as a change from their drab environment in the back streets of London, and other industrial towns. In the beginning, it was a labour of love and as such, it has remained. There is no reward, except the satisfaction of doing something for those less fortunate than ourselves. It started in a simple and very personal way, just by having a few poor children down to stay on the farm of the house (Frensham Place) in which we lived, and, for greater numbers, arranging with the cooperation of what was then the Waifs and Strays Society to send parties of London children for a day's outing to Epping Forest [in Essex]. These country outings for those condemned to the slum life of our big cities, were soon extended, but for a

long time visits to Loughton (in the Epping Forest district of Essex) marked the opening of the Fresh Air Fund holiday season.

Sir Neville also described how, as the years went by, 'a number of distinguished people graced the occasion by their presence, including members of our Royal Family'.[1]

In the April 1892 edition of *Pearson's Weekly*, Pearson himself declared, in respect of the Fresh Air Fund:

> We are very anxious to make arrangements which, during the coming summer, will result in many poor London children having a breath of pure country air which to most of them is such a rarity. We believe that we shall be able to arrange for children to have a day in the country within a radius of 20 miles of London for 9d [ninepence] a head. This sum including railway fares and a supply of good food. Now what we have set our hearts on is to raise enough money to enable us to send a party of 2,000 children away for a day's outing every weekday between June 13th and September 17th!

He suggested to those of his readers who were planning their own holidays, that they might wish to

> Remember these little ones into whose lives so little pleasure enters, and spare from the sum you are setting aside for your own enjoyment enough to secure, for a few of them, a day's release from the grime and dullness of their squalid surroundings – a day of pleasure in the fresh air and sunshine, the green fields and brightness, that to them will be a veritable glimpse of paradise.

The outcome was that

> A generous public immediately forwarded subscriptions in response to the announcement to such an extent that the first party of 2,000 children were taken to Snaresbrook on the outskirts of Epping Forest on June 15th 1892.[2]

Shortly after the founding of the Fresh Air Fund, Pearson collaborated with John Kirk, General Secretary of the Ragged School Union, whose organisation had been running a small holiday fund in London for several years. Founded by the 7th Earl of Shaftesbury in 1884, the Ragged School Union's purpose was to create free schools for poor children throughout the country. In 1914, it was renamed The Shaftesbury Society, the aim of which was to support people with disability or on low income.

When Pearson founded the *Daily Express* in 1900, and subsequently took control of a number of other newspapers, he was able to use these publications – in addition to *Pearson's Weekly* – as a vehicle to advertise his Fresh Air Fund. He also enlisted the help of some of the most powerful and influential people of the day, among them Scottish businessman and philanthropist Sir Thomas Lipton; Australian operatic soprano Dame Nellie Melba; novelist Marie Corelli; Scottish statesman and philosopher the Right Honourable A. J. Balfour; English writer Rudyard Kipling; and the Bishop of Winchester. Also, English actress Gladys Cooper and English soldier and founder of the Scout Movement, General Baden-Powell – about whom more later.

By the year 1901, no less than 29 cities and towns in the United Kingdom had been incorporated into Pearson's Fresh Air Fund – each with its own local committee – and by the end of the first decade of the Fund's life 767,625 children had enjoyed a day out in the countryside. So successful was Pearson at fundraising for his new venture that by the end of July 1893, sufficient money was available to hold additional excursions to Pollard's Hill, Norbury – a beauty spot in north Surrey.

Pearson revealed just how much he empathised with these 'thousands of little children in our great cities who never see the country and never breathe the fresh air', when he wrote:

> The scent of hayfields, the shaded hedgerows, diversified with fragrant flowers, the peaceful woodlands, are all unknown to them. They never bathe their feet in the running stream, nor see the butterflies, nor hear the birds singing. They do not know the joy of living. How good a thing it was to hear the laughter of the city children at play in the meadows and woods – to let them feast 'al fresco' to their small hearts' content on wholesome country fare.

Yet he was not satisfied with the children having just one day's holiday. 'I SHOULD LIKE EVERY CHILD TO BE AWAY FOR AT LEAST TWO WEEKS', he wrote.[3]

In 1910, HM King George V assented to become the Fresh Air Fund's Patron. On 1 March, the Fund was incorporated into a company, and on 1 April it held its first General Meeting, with Pearson as President. That year, declared Pearson, had been

… noteworthy for the number of crippled children for whom a holiday has been arranged … the fund this year took from town to country a little army of 6,000 cripples, and there also went, for the fresh air holidays 1,000 blind children.[4]

In fact, in 1910, 94,117 children from London and 131,550 children from the larger provincial towns had a day in the countryside, and 1,500 children from London and 2,620 children from the provinces had a full fortnight's holiday.[5] Also in that year, the Fund was registered under the Companies Act and of its seven trustees, all but one was connected with the newspaper industry.

4

Pearson Remarries:
Frensham Place

In 1897, Pearson, now a 31-year-old widower and a wealthy man, married Ethel Maud, daughter of William John Fraser Esquire, of 'Cromartie', Herne Bay, Kent. By her he had a son, Neville Arthur, born 13 February 1898. The couple set up home at Frensham Place in Farnham, Surrey. Neville did not follow in the footsteps of his father and grandfather by going to Winchester. Instead, he went to Eton College. Here, showing the same athletic prowess as his paternal forebears, he excelled at cricket, becoming captain of the First XI in 1916 and also at fives, winning the school competition two years in a row.

Built by a French architect, Frensham Place, an elegant mansion – which included a ballroom – was originally the home of the Seilern family. The great art collector Count Antoine Seilern was born here in 1901 and this is where he spent his early years. The Frensham Estate of 120 acres included a farm, granary, orchard, kitchen gardens, park, stables, pleasure gardens, a lake and pine woods. Here, Pearson laid out an 18-hole golf course, established an indoor riding school and converted part of the stables into an aviary in which he kept his collection of rare birds. He also kept bees, and planted lavender bushes in profusion to provide them with nectar.

As Pearson commuted back and forth to London to work, a colleague of his, who preferred to remain anonymous, declared that Pearson

… never wasted a moment of the long train journey to Town [London]. When the return journey was made in the dark he would still work on manuscripts and proofs, using a little lamp fastened in the buttonhole of his coat, so that he could read.

In his hours of leisure, said the colleague, he was equally strenuous, and was

… always ready to take up something new. When he began keeping horses, he started at once to drive a tandem and a four-in-hand without any previous experience. He trusted to his own judgment and skill. His only accident, it is recorded, was when the front part of a wagonette broke away from the body of the carriage and Mr Pearson, who was driving a spirited pair of horses, refusing to let go of the reins, was dragged a long distance down the road. For a time he was laid up for his injuries, but he was compensated for his inaction by thinking that the horses had not got away from him!

Pearson enjoyed caravanning holidays and collecting ivory carvings. However, said the colleague, he cared little for art or music.[1] He also enjoyed a round of golf, but sadly, in the words of journalist, art collector and historian Bernard Falk: 'It was while playing golf at Frensham near Farnham, that he first realised that he was going blind. He could no longer see the ball.'[2]

At Frensham Place, the Pearsons enjoyed entertaining their London friends, one of whom was the Scottish playwright and novelist J. M. Barrie. Barrie had started life as a journalist and was now an author. His books were characterised by whimsical humour, with allusions to the darker sides of life. In the grounds of Frensham Place, Pearson built an elaborate tree house, and it is believed that this may have inspired Barrie when he wrote his dramatic fantasy *Peter Pan* (1904). In the story, Wendy, having been injured soon after her arrival in 'Neverland', is taken to a little house built by Peter. (Such houses subsequently became known as 'Wendy Houses'.)

When motor cars became popular, Pearson was only interested in the high-powered variety, which he drove with 'characteristic recklessness'.[3] Basil Gotto described how Pearson had offered to drive him home to London from the Sandown Park racecourse – of which both men were members – and in doing so, gave him a 'great fright'. Gotto:

In the matter of speed, Pearson habitually flaunted the law, and we travelled at 40 miles an hour. I held on to my seat, my hat, my breath, and knew my last hour had come, and I should never see my home again.[4]

Like the cars that he drove, Pearson himself appeared to be supercharged. He spoke in short, clipped sentences, leaving out unnecessary words. He was always to the point, often in a hurry and dispensed with frills. However, this 'abrupt, staccato way of talking', says Sidney Dark, was a shield which he 'carefully cultivated to protect himself from his own impulsive good nature'.[5]

Such frantic activity must eventually take its toll, as his anonymous colleague indicated.

In those early days he almost invariably fell asleep immediately after dinner. Even if he had guests he would often vanish to a deckchair or hammock. There was nothing he disliked more than being aroused to go to bed.[6]

5

Pearson and Grant Allen

A particular delight for Pearson was to drive the 8 miles to Hindhead – his eyesight had not yet deteriorated enough to prevent him from doing this – and visit his friend Grant Allen, who was eighteen years his senior. Allen was a Canadian writer who came to Hindhead in 1893 and built a house, 'The Croft' there. When his life is examined, it is easy to see why Pearson found him such good company.

Allen was a socialist, a Darwinist, and (despite the fact that his father was a Protestant minister) an agnostic. He wrote prodigiously and in this he was a true polymath. No subject appeared to escape his notice and he was regarded as a pre-eminent populariser of modern science. Allen shared Pearson's love of nature and amongst his titles are to be found *Dissecting a Daisy*, *The Origin of Flora*, *Speckled Trout*, *Flowers and their Pedigrees*, and *A Naturalist's Year*. Allen was also the editor of English naturalist and clergyman Gilbert White's *History of Selbourne*. Allen's more esoteric works include *How Flowers appeal to Human Aesthetic Sensibilities* and *Butterfly Psychology*.

Between 1884 and 1899 – the year of his death – Allen wrote in the region of 30 novels, some of which were science fiction. His avant-garde novel *The Woman who Did*, written in 1895, which told the story of a woman of independent means who had a child out of wedlock, aroused a great deal of controversy.

Allen shared Pearson's fascination with the human mind and the latter would undoubtedly have been intrigued by the ideas expressed in *The Evolution of the Idea of God: An Enquiry into the Origins of Religions* (1897), and *Nation-Making: A Theory of National Characters* (1878). Pearson's interest in the occult (which will be discussed in more detail later) found resonance in Allen's *Pausodyne* (1881), which was concerned with the creation of an analgesic that brings about a catatonic trance resulting in suspended animation, and *My New Year's Eve amongst the Mummies* (which Allen wrote under the pseudonym 'J. Arbuthnot Wilson') in which the narrator stumbles across the entrance to a pyramid, and inside he discovers a pharaoh and his court enjoying a meal. These are mummies which come to life for a day and a night once in every 1,000 years. This latter title was published by *Pearson's Weekly* in 1893.

At Hindhead, Allen was a neighbour of writer Arthur Conan Doyle. Doyle and Pearson would undoubtedly have met, the former also being greatly interested in the occult, for in 1897, three of Doyle's 'Captain Sharkey' pirate stories were featured in *Pearson's Weekly*.

6

Pearson the Newspaper Proprietor: Tariff Reform

Having witnessed the success of the *Daily Mail*, founded by Lord Northcliffe in 1896, Pearson had the idea of creating a newspaper of his own. In order for the launch to go well, he was anxious to obtain an item of news which was both 'fresh and striking.' He therefore sent for 22-year-old Hesketh V. H. Prichard.

Prichard was the son of Hesketh Brodrick Prichard, an officer in the British Army, who had died of typhoid fever at the age of 25 whilst on active service in Afghanistan in 1876. He was a Fellow of both the Royal Geographical Society and the Zoological Society. He was also a writer, who, in 1897, Pearson had commissioned, together with his mother Kate, to contribute some ghost stories for *Pearson's Magazine*. This they did under the pseudonyms 'E. & H. Heron'. The stories – of which there were twelve – featured the 'psychic detective' Flaxman Low.

Prichard volunteered to travel to and explore the Caribbean island of Haiti:

No white man had crossed Haiti, or indeed, had travelled into the interior for a hundred years, since the blacks in 1803 revolted against the French settlers and massacred them. [To date] All that had come to the outer world from Haiti were rumours ... of snake-worship and poisonings, human sacrifice and cannibalism.[1]

Pearson agreed to the idea, and Prichard arrived in Haiti in November 1899.

Publication of the *Daily Express*, which cost one halfpenny per copy (and into which the *Morning Herald*, which Pearson had acquired in 1898, was merged) duly commenced in April 1900. Pearson was its first editor, his office being at 8 Tudor Street in the City. The battle-cry of the *Daily Express* was: 'Truth and Right, Independence, Sympathy, Justice for All.'

The front page of the very first issue of the *Daily Express* contained an invitation to the reader to enjoy the first of a series of articles by Mr Hesketh Prichard concerning his visit to 'Hayti [Haiti], the Black Republic'. Readers were assured that Prichard's revelations in regard to the island would 'undoubtedly afford a world sensation'.

The front page also carried an apology. Although orders had been received for 1,500,000 copies of the *Daily Express*, 'it is an absolute impossibility', said the management, 'to supply this unprecedented and entirely unforeseen demand, but we are doing our best'.

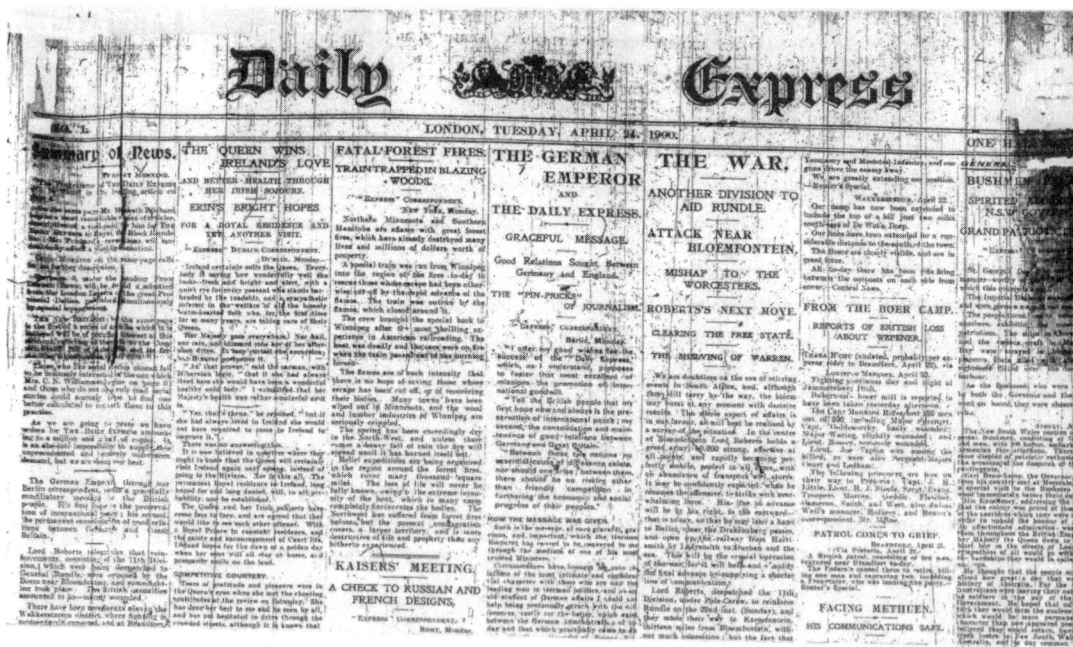

The *Daily Express*: the first ever issue, Tuesday 24 April 1900. Photo: British Library.

The front page was otherwise devoted entirely to news of the British Empire, and to the relating of a personal message sent to that newspaper by the German Emperor Wilhelm II (known as 'The Kaiser'). It read as follows:

I offer my good wishes for the success of the 'Daily Express,' which, as I understand, proposes to foster that most excellent of missions, the promotion of international goodwill.

Tell the British people that my first hope, now and always, is the preservation of international peace; my second, the consolidation and maintenance of good relations between Germany and Great Britain.

Between these two nations no essential cause of difference exists, nor should one arise between them. There should be no rivalry, other than friendly competition in furthering the economic and social progress of their peoples.

As for the British Empire, the *Daily Express* appears to have had correspondents everywhere. There was news from Natal, Orange Free State, and Cape Colony on how the Boer War was progressing, and an indication that British General, Lord Roberts, with his army of 50,000 men, was preparing to strike at the Boers, 'with overwhelming force'. Meanwhile, in the Australian colony of New South Wales, the 'New South Wales Imperial Bushmen' were preparing to embark for South Africa. This was one of a number of regiments raised in the Australian colonies in response to a request by the British Government for 'hardy bushmen' who could ride, shoot, and navigate their way through the bush, in order to use guerrilla tactics against the Boers and thereby beat them at their own game.

The *Daily Express's* 'War Editor' in Cape Town was Fletcher Robinson, a friend of Arthur Conan Doyle. When, in 1899, Pearson recalled Robinson to London, he offered Robinson's post to artist and sculptor Basil Gotto. Born in 1866 in Highgate, London, Gotto had studied painting at the Académie Julian in Paris, and in 1887 had entered the Royal Academy (R. A.) as a sculptor. For the next few years, he specialised mainly in creating marble or bronze portrait busts, but he also produced statues of figures from Greek mythology and painted portraits. He exhibited regularly at the R. A.

Gotto described Pearson as 'an unusual type for a [news] paper proprietor. He was a highly educated man with a sensibility which he afterwards proved.' Pearson, said Gotto, demonstrated this sensibility on more than one occasion. For example, during the Boxer Revolution of 1899–90 (the uprising of Chinese nationalists against foreign influence in that country) a report came in to say that all foreign ambassadors in China had been murdered. Despite the fact that this report came from 'our correspondent – a most trustworthy Mandarin', Pearson decided not to publish it, as it was uncorroborated, believing: 'It can only give pain [i.e. to the friends and relations of the ambassadors who had been allegedly murdered,] and after all, it may not be true.'

Pearson demonstrated his willingness to adopt new ideas, even to the point of eccentricity. On the occasion of his being told by a doctor, during an influenza epidemic, that the best preventative for this disease was eucalyptus oil, he acted upon the information with energy:

> As soon as he arrived at his office next day he bought all the eucalyptus oil he could lay his hands on, and fifty helpers were put to work squirting it through scent sprays onto each copy of the paper as it came off the machines.[2]

A notable contributor to the *Daily Express* was the famous athlete and sportsman Charles Burgess ('CB') Fry (born in 1872.) Fry's many and varied achievements included equalling the World Long Jump Record of 23ft 6½in in June 1893, playing football for England and captaining his home country at cricket. He went on to become a sports journalist, and in 1904 created *C. B. Fry's Magazine*, which was devoted to physical culture and health. For 40 years he served as Director of the training ship *Mercury* at Hamble, Hampshire – a nautical school designed to prepare boys for service in the Royal Navy. Fry contributed a series of signed articles on sporting matters to the *Daily Express*, one of which was entitled 'The Decline and Fall of English Football'.

Fry paints an amusing portrait of Pearson at work, where he lived, 'in a whirl of hustle which to him appeared to be the essence of efficiency', noting he 'made a point of being an immediate yes–or–no man'. All submissions to the *Daily Express* were examined by Pearson, and if the paragraphs which were contained in them were deemed by him to be too long, he would divide them up into smaller but equal portions, as if with the aid of a ruler. To the writer, said Fry, this could be 'quite startling'.[3]

On 22 January 1901, the energetic and enthusiastic Pearson was almost responsible for the demise of his own newspaper. The long reign of the sovereign Queen Victoria was coming to a close, and she was gravely ill at Osborne House – her royal residence on the Isle of Wight – and her death was expected imminently. Gotto said:

> It was for that moment that Pearson made his preparations. When the Great Queen passed away, a handkerchief was to be waved from a window in Osborne, [whereupon] a pigeon was to be released for flight to Portsmouth [on the mainland], and thence a telephone to London would launch upon the Empire myriads of cables giving the momentous news.

However, only five minutes after the plan had been executed and the pigeon released, Pearson received a telephone call: 'News uncertain, detain cables.' It is not difficult to imagine the condition of Pearson, who, according to Gotto was 'in perfect agony', fearing that the *Daily Express* would surely, 'expire from ridicule'. Another ten 'interminable minutes' passed before further news of the Queen arrived. Yes, she had indeed passed away, 'and Pearson and his paper lived again'.[4]

It was as a result of a meeting between Pearson and Conservative politician Joseph Chamberlain (Colonial Secretary 1895–1903, when he resigned his office) in July 1903, that the Tariff Reform League was created, with Pearson as its Chairman. Its objective was to establish a single trading bloc within the British Empire, and to impose tariffs on goods entering it from the rest of the world. There were those, however, who feared that the result of such import duties would be a rise in the price of food. Because of the vigour which Pearson applied to the cause of Tariff Reform, Chamberlain nicknamed him 'The Great Hustler'. The issue, however, divided the Conservative Party and was a major factor in its landslide defeat by the Liberals in the election of January 1906.

In 1903, Pearson acquired the *St James's Gazette*. In 1904, he purchased *The Standard* and its sister newspaper *The Evening Standard,* which he amalgamated with the *St James's Gazette*, and changed the stance of both newspapers from a Conservative one to a Liberal one. However sales declined, and in 1910 he sold them both. He also made an unsuccessful attempt to take over *The Times*, but did acquire a controlling interest in many provincial newspapers, including the *Birmingham Daily Gazette*, the *Leicester Evening News*, the *North Mail*, the *Midland Express* and the *Newcastle Weekly Leader*.

Over the course of the next few years, Pearson's eyesight continued to deteriorate, the condition having been diagnosed as glaucoma – a disease in which the pressure within the eyeballs rises unduly and destroys the optic nerves. In March 1908, he underwent surgery (today, glaucoma would have been treated, initially, with pressure-relieving eye drops). The operation, performed by Mr Robert Doyne, was not a lasting success, and soon Pearson was unable to see well enough either to read or write. Two years later, he took his wife Ethel and their children to Switzerland, determined that if blindness were to overtake him, which seemed inevitable, then he would first see as much of that beautiful country as he could.

As time went by, Pearson found himself devoting an increasing amount of time to his pursuits at Frensham Place, and less to his business empire. He enjoyed riding in the woods, driving horses, and boating on and swimming in the lake. This life of idyllic rusticity, however, was interspersed with sporadic episodes of furious activity.

7

Pearson and the Search for the Giant Sloth

At the end of the nineteenth and beginning of the twentieth century, rumours began to emanate from South America, and in particular from the region of Patagonia – part of which lies in Argentina and part in Chile – about the possible existence of a large, hairy, bear-like creature known to the ancients, but now believed to be extinct. This was the megatherium, or giant ground sloth (a relation of the mylodon, or small ground sloth, which exists today).

In anticipation of achieving a great scoop for his newspaper, in late 1900 Pearson sent again for Hesketh Prichard, who was commissioned to travel to Patagonia in the hope that he would discover a living example of this creature. In Prichard's words:

> Mr Pearson, the proprietor of the *Daily Express*, most generously financed the Expedition in the interests of science, and entrusted me with the task of sifting all the evidence for or against the chances of survival [of the megatherium] obtainable on the spot.[1]

The *Daily Express* edition of 22 June 1900, bore the following headline:

GIANT SLOTH OF PATAGONIA
A NEW 'EXPRESS' SCIENTIFIC EXPEDITION

In search of the extraordinary animal, described in the following report of
a lecture delivered last night, the 'Express' is sending a special expedition
to Patagonia under the command of Mr Hesketh Prichard, whose brilliant
letters from the black republic of Hayti we recently published.

Upon what evidence were the rumours of the creature's existence based?
As author Gavin Menzies points out, a 'dog-headed' creature (the shape
of a human being, but stockier, with large head, elongated nose and jaw,
and short tail) appeared in a Chinese book entitled *The Illustrated Record of
Strange Countries* (*I Yü Thu Chih*), published in 1430, author unknown. Of
its 132 illustrations, there are plants, animals and people from practically
every part of the globe. The creature, it says, was 'found two years and nine
month's journey west of China'.[2]

The Illustrated Record of Strange Countries was undoubtedly published as the
result of several voyages undertaken by the Chinese in the 1420s. The most
notable of these being the epic 2-year voyage of four huge Chinese fleets
which set sail from Beijing on 8 March 1421, on the orders of Emperor Zhu
Di. The fleets were 'to proceed all the way to the end of the earth', which
they did, achieving the extraordinary feat of circumnavigating the larger
portion of all the continents.

One of these fleets, commanded by Admiral Zhou Man, is known to
have crossed the Indian Ocean, sailed round the Cape of Good Hope,
travelled northwards to the Cape Verde Islands, then southwards towards
Cape Horn, through what later became known as the Straits of Magellan,
before sailing on up the western coast of South America and returning
home via the Pacific Ocean. In other words, this Chinese fleet preceded
that of Portuguese navigator Ferdinand Magellan – who sailed through the
straits (which subsequently bore his name) in October 1520 – by almost a
century. Also, as Magellan's fleet appeared to know precisely where it was
going, it is possible that it was using charts based on those drawn up by the
navigators who had sailed with Admiral Zhou Man.

In 1513, Ottoman-Turkish admiral and cartographer Piri Reis produced
a map of the world, which, as he himself admitted, was based on at least
20 other maps which had preceded it. On the South American portion of
the Piri Reis map, in the region of what is now known as Patagonia, five
creatures are depicted: a deer, a guanaco (a member of the camel family),
a mountain lion, a bearded man and a dog-headed creature similar to that
in *The Illustrated Record of Strange Countries*. The implication is that the

Chinese were aware of the existence of such a creature as long ago as the early 1420s.

The Piri Reis map of Patagonia also included two notes, which were of great significance as far as the dog-headed creature was concerned. One stated that: 'in this place there are … wild beasts of this sort',[3] and the other that 'these wild beasts attain a length of seven spans [a span being the distance between the tips of the thumb and little finger of the outstretched hand]'.[4] In other words, the creature was of similar size to an adult human being.

Finally, the statement that the discovery was made after a 'two years and nine month's journey' from China, correlates with the fact that this is the length of time that it would have taken Admiral Zhou Man's fleet to journey to that region. (Menzies has suggested that the Chinese may have taken one or more megatheriae back to China to present to the Emperor for his zoo; this being their custom in respect of all rare or newly-discovered creatures.)

Was Pearson aware of the existence of this ancient book and map? Almost certainly not. *The Illustrated Record of Strange Countries* which was donated to the University of Cambridge in the late nineteenth century, is unique, and the Piri Reis map was only discovered in 1929, when the Palace of Topkapi in Istanbul, Turkey, was being converted into a museum. There was, however, more recent evidence for the existence of the dog-headed creature of which Pearson *was* almost certainly aware.

In 1831, more than four centuries after Chinese Admiral Zhou Man's epic voyage, English naturalist Charles Darwin, travelled on the ship HMS *Beagle,* captained by Robert Fitzroy, whose task it was to make a scientific survey of South American waters. Darwin would not return until 1836. The expedition made several visits to Punta Alta on Argentina's Atlantic coast, where many bones were to be found wedged in the cliffs. On one visit Darwin found an almost complete skeleton of a megatherium, which he presented to Dr Richard Owen, Conservator of London's Hunterian Museum (named after Scottish physiologist and surgeon John Hunter). Owen not only confirmed the identity of the skeleton, he reconstructed it and displayed it in his museum raised up on its hind legs, grasping a tree trunk with its forelegs.

It was clear that megatherium was one of the largest mammals ever to walk the earth – weighing as much as an African bull elephant, in excess of 4 tons. It was bear-like in appearance, with an elongated nose and curved claws. By standing on its hind legs – when it attained the height of about 20 feet (far in excess of the 'seven spans' indicated on the Piri Reis map) – it could use these claws to pull down the branches of trees, in order to reach the leaves upon which it fed. It also ate grasses.

In *The Origin of Species*, Darwin wrote:

> It may be asked in ridicule whether I suppose that the megatherium and other allied huge monsters, which formerly lived in South America, have left behind them the sloth, armadillo, and anteater as their degenerate descendants. This cannot for an instant be admitted. These huge animals have become wholly extinct, and have left no progeny.[5]

Would Pearson's expedition prove Darwin's last sentence wrong by finding a living megatherium? (Darwinism tells us that he could be wrong in the first assertion, concerning degenerate descendants!)

In 1895, local sheep farmer Herman Eberhardt discovered the skin of what he believed to be a sea mammal at Last Hope Inlet, near the southernmost tip of South America in Chilean Patagonia. He hung it on a tree and thought no more about it. Two years later, it was discovered by an Argentinian naturalist and explorer Dr F. Perito Moreno, who was conducting a survey of the boundary line between Chile and Argentina. Moreno was told that this was only a fragment of a larger piece of skin which had been discovered in a cave in the neighbouring hills. He expressed the opinion that the skin belonged to a pampean mylodon (i.e. whose habitat was the pampas.) However, Moreno was puzzled by how well the piece of skin was preserved, and he attributed this to the fact that in the cave where it was found, the atmosphere would have been dry. Moreno was correct, for in the dry and excessively cold atmosphere which pertained, the skin had become mummified. This had prevented any significant decomposition.[6] Moreno took the fragment of skin to the British Museum in London, where it was identified as that of a megatherium. Subsequently, the skin was shown – by Carbon-14 dating – to be in the region of 5,000 years old.

The cave in question was subsequently excavated further by geologist Dr Rudolph Hauthal of Argentina's La Plata Museum of Natural History near Buenos Aires. Buried in the earth of its floor were found the bones of several megatheriae, together with a thick deposit of their excrement and 'an extensive accumulation of cut hay'. This led Hauthal to conclude that this cave was an old corral in which the megatheriae had been kept and fed by man (though for what purpose is not stated).[7]

Finally, in Britain, Professor Ray E. Lancaster, Director of the British Museum of Natural History, South Kensington (which had taken custody of the skin) set the whole country ablaze with 'giant sloth fever' when, in a lecture to the Zoological Society on 21 June 1900, he declared tantalisingly: 'It is quite possible – I don't want to say more than that – that he [the megatherium] still exists in some of the mountainous regions of Patagonia.'[8]

This idea was reinforced by Argentinian animal collector Carlos Armeghino (brother of Dr Florentino Armeghino, paleontologist and Deputy Director of the La Plata Museum) who expressed the opinion that the animal was still living in Patagonia; the local Indians having told him of: 'a vast mysterious beast said by them to haunt the distant lagoons and forests of the unexplored regions near the Andes [and] to roam the pampas'. So great was its strength that it could 'seize a horse in its claws. In size, it far exceeded any creature they knew of'.[9]

To return to the expedition, sponsored by Pearson and led by Prichard, which consisted of eight men, 60 horses, a waggon and a boat: having arrived at Puerto Madryn, Argentina, in September 1900, it set out on the 15th of that month and travelled westwards towards the Andes mountains.

Prichard kept a diary, extracts from which were sent back to England at regular intervals to be printed in the *Daily Express* and read avidly by its readers. When high in the Chilean Andes, north of Lake Argentino, he discovered a lake, he named it Lake Pearson. However, despite journeying 1,750 miles overland, he found no trace of his quarry. He therefore set sail for home from Punta Arenas in the far south of Chile in late May 1901.

Prichard amassed a wealth of information about the topography of Patagonia, its peoples, its flora (156 species of plants were collected and catalogued) and its fauna. He also brought back with him a unique collection of photographs. On his return to England he presented (on Pearson's behalf) the skin of a puma which he had acquired to the Natural History Museum, where it was examined by Oldfield Thomas, Fellow of the Royal Society. Thomas declared that the skin, which was 'remarkably unlike any known form of puma,' was of a sub-species of *Felis concolor* (pumas being known locally in Patagonia as lions), saying: 'In commemoration of Mr Pearson's scientific spirit in sending out the expedition ... I would propose to call it *Felis concolor Pearsoni*.'[10]

'Pearson's puma' differed from other sub-species of *Felis concolor* – now named *Puma concolor* – in that it was 'clay-colour in hue, thick and sturdy in build, with comparatively short limbs and tail'.[11] *Puma concolor Pearsoni* is now one of 29 recognised sub-species of the puma, or mountain lion.

Was this the end of the story? Perhaps, perhaps not, for as Prichard remarked, there were

> … hundreds of square miles of dense forest still unexplored along the whole length of the Patagonian Andes. I do not undertake to declare positively, that no such animal exists in some unknown and hidden spot among their recesses.[12]

Pearson and his *Daily Express* newspaper were not the only beneficiaries of the publicity gained by Prichard's expedition. Author Arthur Conan Doyle's imagination was also gripped by the story, which he used as the basis for part of his novel *The Lost World*.

Prichard's work for Pearson was not yet done, for in early 1902, he was sent to Ireland 'in order to try to discover the causes of the so-called "unrest" in that country'.[13]

8

C. Arthur Pearson Ltd: Pearson the Author: Pearson and the Occult

Pearson had always been a writer, even in his youth, when he had written and had published articles on subjects such as birds (including American songbirds), trees, snails and spiders – nature being a favourite subject of his.[1]

In the early 1900s Pearson's company, C. Arthur Pearson Ltd, published a series of guide books under the title of *Pearson's Gossipy Guides*. They included, in 1901, *Pearson's Gossipy Guide to Glasgow, the Clyde District, and the International Exhibition of 1901*. Others featured the cities of Edinburgh, London and Paris; the County of Devonshire; and the English Lake District (complete with illustrations and maps). Pearsons also published historical novels, such as George Griffith's *The Virgin of the Sun: A Tale of the Conquest of Peru*, and *The Rose of Judah: A Tale of the Captivity*, together with science fiction novels, such as Austin Fryer's *The Devil and the Inventor*, in which an impoverished inventor enlists the help of the devil.

The motto of *Pearson's Weekly* was 'To Interest, to Elevate, to Amuse,' and this ethos applied equally to a series of booklets published by C. Arthur Pearson Ltd, entitled *Handbooks on Useful Hobbies*, or *Handbooks of General Information*. The aim was to provide a diverse range of titles that would appeal to a wide range of people. Titles were produced in hardback and priced at between one shilling and two shillings and threepence (2/3d), with an extra threepence payable if the customer required it to be sent 'post free'.

The practically-minded could choose from *Metalwork; Photography for Beginners; Model-making; Carpentry and Cabinet-making.* For the sporting there was *Rowing and Sculling; Boxing; Practical Fishing; The Game of Billiards; Cricket.* For the housewife: *Dainty Dishes – Cold Meat and How To Disguise It; Our Food and Drinks; Vegetarian Cookery; Little Economies and How to Practise Them; Plain Needlework.* For the gardener: *Small Gardens and How to Make the Most of Them; Roses and How to Grow Them; Greenhouses and How to Manage Them.* For those interested in animals and pets: *Rabbit-keeping For Pleasure and Profit; Poultry-keeping; The Dog in Health and Disease; Cage and Singing Birds.* For the would-be conjurer: *Card tricks; Conjuring with Coins;* and *Magic Made Easy.*

Courting couples could avail themselves of *The Lovers' Guide;* whereas for the prospective parent there was *Names for Baby.* In the unhappy event of sickness striking the family, or in order to ward it off, the following titles – all written by qualified physicians – were available: *Infectious Diseases and How to Prevent Them; The Mother's Guide to the Care of Children in Sickness and Health; Every Woman her Own Doctor; Home Nursing;* and *Indigestion and How to Cure It.*

For those anxious to succeed in life there were two titles, written by Pearson's managing director Peter Keary himself: *The Secret of Success;* and *Get On or Get Out.* The upper or aspiring classes might benefit from a perusal of *Servants have their Duties; The Drawing Room Entertainer; The Art of Correct Letter-Writing for Men and Women on All Occasions; Etiquette for Women; Etiquette for Men;* and *The Etiquette of Engagement & Marriage.*

Close to Pearson's own heart were books on the following subjects: *How and What to Dance; Pearson's Light Car Handbook – How to Choose and Drive a Car;* and *Golf for Beginners.*

Interestingly, there was a large selection of books on the occult (defined as concerned with the supernatural, mystical, magical)[2] including *Hands and How to Read Them* by E. René; *Heads and How to Read Them* by Stackpool E. O'Dell; *Astrology – How to Make and Read your own Horoscope* by 'Old Moore'; and *Consult the Oracle, Or How to Read the Future.*

Even more revealing, four of C. Arthur Pearson's books on the occult were written by Pearson himself, all in 1902, and all under the pseudonym 'Professor P. R. S. Foli'. These were *Pearson's Dream Book; Pearson's Fortune Teller; Fortune Telling By Cards;* and *Handwriting as an Index to Character.*

Pearson gives the impression that these four books were written purely for the amusement of the 'inquirer' and yet, in the same breath, he presents them as works worthy of serious consideration. So why was this energetic, able, practical and seemingly level-headed man, who had created a business empire out of nothing, so interested in the occult, and do his four books on the subject give any insight into how his own mind may have been working?

Pearson's Dream Book

This is concerned not only with dreams but also with 'messages of fate' and with omens. The subject is introduced with a quotation from the Biblical prophet Job: 'In a dream, in a vision of the night, when deep sleep falleth upon men, in slumberings upon the bed, then He openeth the ears of men, and sealeth their instruction.' These words, Pearson says, 'are confirmed by daily experience. 'With full confidence … we claim that a supernatural agency is at work to shape our dreams.'

Under the heading 'What are Dreams?' Pearson affirms:

> It must be a very incredulous and unscientific mind that refuses to give due weight to all the evidences we possess from reliable sources, in proof that dreams are sent as direct warning, revelation, or comfort to mortals in danger, doubt, or distress.

The interpretation of dreams, he says, was a 'recognised profession among the Ancient Greeks', and he goes on to quote what they and the Romans, and more recently, such eminent people as William Shakespeare, Sir Thomas Brown, Joseph Addison and John Bunyan have said about dreams. To Pearson, the opinions of such people were not to be ignored.

He divides dreams into three main types:

1. *The Dream Proper*, or *Vision*, which tells us the truth during our sleep under accepted figures or symbols.
2. *The Oracle*, which is a revelation sent to us in our dreams to clear up some mystery or doubt.
3. *The Warning* which is intended to put us on guard against some malign influence or danger.

It was possible to interpret dreams, said Pearson by using 'the wonderful Table of Magic Cyphers, which Napoleon had consulted at any crisis of his career'.

In his dream book, Pearson purports to offer the reader a method of interpreting the meaning of his or her dream. In so doing, he implies that he himself may believe in the possibility of dream interpretation. Before enquiring as to why this should be so, it is instructive to examine his three other books about the occult.

Pearson's Fortune Teller

Pearson again invokes the experiences of the ancients in order to add weight to his arguments. The Ancient Egyptians, Greeks, Romans and Celts were in the habit of studying the stars for omens and signs, in the hope of acquiring a fore-knowledge of events. He stated: 'Even in the twentieth century the majority of us are not proof against the fascination of those means by which we hope to obtain a glimpse of what lies in the future.' What could be more unequivocal than this statement of Pearson's, which shows that he shared in this fascination. However, on a less serious note, he expresses the hope that 'amusement' will accompany the study of his book's pages, together with 'gratification'.

Pearson discusses 'Planchette, the Mysterious Writing Board,' and poses the question: 'What power causes this simple contrivance to move and write intelligible things which are often extraordinarily prophetic?' Does the explanation 'lie within some undiscovered part of ourselves, or is there some outside influence of which those who use Planchette are only the medium? The reader must form his own conclusion.' In succeeding chapters, he goes on to deal with subjects such as cartomancy (or card-reading), astrology, crystal-gazing, palmistry, psychic power, and the significance of the shapes of tea leaves left behind in a cup after drinking.

Handwriting as an Index to Character

Pearson describes how graphology (the study of handwriting) can be used to deduce a person's 'temperament or constitution', 'matrimonial adaptability' and 'fitness for occupations in life.' The handwriting of different nationalities, says Pearson, is an indication of national character. The French, for example, showing 'extreme sensibility and proneness to take offence at trifles', whereas American handwriting reflects that nation's 'go-ahead, speculative character'.

Fortune Telling by Cards
(A booklet which has remained in print up until the present time)

Here, Pearson affirms that cartomancy (the telling of fortunes by studying and interpreting a 'random' selection of playing cards), 'has swayed the human mind from prehistoric times right down to this twentieth century of ours'. And he makes a comment which, perhaps more than any other, reveals what may have been going through his mind at this particular time:

> There is a vein of superstition in every human heart, and many men who have played a great part in the world's history have not been too ashamed to seek help from occultists, when the tangle of life seemed too involved for them to unravel with the ordinary means at their disposal.

From his four titles on occult subjects – written by him when he was aged 36 – what can be deduced about Pearson himself? The books certainly indicate that their author had an enquiring mind, but did this son of a clergyman really believe in supernatural power?

For all his outward self-confidence, Pearson realised that a time bomb was ticking away inside him, his eyesight was gradually deteriorating and short of a miracle, the likelihood was that he would soon lose his sight altogether. Despite being the son of a clergyman, he appears not to have derived solace from Christianity, for in his book *Victory over Blindness*, there is little mention of religion. Also, when his horoscope was read and the astrologer made the comment: 'I do not think spirituality has a marked place in his composition,' Pearson, (according to Sidney Dark) concurred with the astrologer's conclusions.[3]

Did Pearson's undoubted interest in the occult arise from a desire to discover what his own future held in store for him? Was he, in reality, an anxious and superstitious man who would clutch at straws in order to find help and comfort? Did this lead him to take what other people said about their dream experiences at face value, to attach undue significance to chance events, such as the upturning of a playing card or domino and to give credence to the prognostications of fortune-tellers? Was his motivation for dabbling in the world of the occult driven, not merely by inquisitiveness, but by anxiety, as he found himself teetering on the edge of a world of total darkness? If this was, indeed, his reason for writing such booklets, then given his situation, perhaps he may be forgiven.

Evidence that Pearson was of a credulous nature is given by Basil Gotto in his *Memoir.* According to Gotto, Pearson's editor, the young and 'stalwart' Fletcher Robinson, decided, against Pearson's advice, to investigate rumours which attached to an Egyptian mummy in the collection at London's British Museum. These rumours, said Gotto, were in circulation well before the discovery by Lord Carnarvon in November 1922, of the tomb of Pharaoh Tutankhamun in Egypt's Valley of the Kings. As far as this mummy was concerned, said Gotto, 'The man who discovered it was said to have died, the porter who moved it broke his leg, in fact every possible calamity followed in its trail.'

Robinson's attempts to 'run these stories to earth', to test their validity were, no doubt, aimed at achieving another scoop for the *Daily Express*. Gotto said that 'Robinson looked on it from the side of an editor ... Pearson ... with just the slightest suspicion of superstition.' The outcome, however, was precisely what Pearson feared it might be. No sooner had Robinson commenced his investigation when he, 'fell ill of diphtheria and died'.[4]

However superstitious Pearson may have been, and whatever knowledge – or expectation – he may have gained from his study of the occult about his own future, the fact remains that the most important and most challenging part of his life was still in front of him. First, however, there were other matters to attend to.

9

Pearson and the Scout Movement

When Robert S. S. Baden-Powell (1857) had the idea of creating the Scout Movement, Pearson was the first person to whom he turned for advice.

Baden-Powell was the sixth son of the Reverend H. G. Baden-Powell, a professor of geometry at Oxford University, who had died when the boy was only three years old. His interest in scouting and woodcraft had begun when he was at school at Charterhouse, Surrey, where he would play in the woods, practise stalking, and catch and cook rabbits in his spare time. On holiday he was equally adventurous: sailing in a yacht round the southern coast of England, and canoeing along the River Thames. He left school to join the army and served with the 13th Hussars in India, Afghanistan and South Africa. It was during the successful defence of Mafeking by the British in the Boer War (when, in October 1899, that town came under a protracted 217-day siege) that Baden-Powell, who commanded the defending detachment of British troops, became famous. He returned to England in 1903 and was appointed Inspector-General of Cavalry. This was when his thoughts turned to the young people of his native land.

In 1904, Baden-Powell was invited by Scottish businessman William A. Smith (later Sir William) to be the inspecting officer for 7,000 members of the Boys' Brigade, who assembled at the Yorkhill Drill Ground in Glasgow. Smith had founded this organisation on 4 October 1883. It emphasised the importance of discipline; encouraged outdoor pursuits, and was a strong advocate of Christian principles. Baden-Powell was impressed by the smart appearance of the participants.

During his time in the army as Major General, Baden-Powell had written several military training manuals including *Reconnaisance and Scouting* (1884), and *Aids to Scouting for NCOs and Men* (1899). Smith now suggested to him that he write a similar manual, designed to be read and used by a younger audience, and he readily agreed.

Due to his army commitments, there was a delay before Baden-Powell was able to embark on the project. However, in 1906, he sent Smith a short article entitled 'Scouting for Boys', which was published that June in the *Boys' Brigade Gazette*. When it was suggested that the Scouts might combine with the Boys' Brigade, Smith declined on the grounds that the make-up of the former did not contain sufficient Christian content.

In July 1906, Baden-Powell visited Pearson at Frensham Place, where the latter 'liked to invite to his week-end parties men of outstanding note in the life of the world'.[1] Pearson's Editor-in-Chief, Percy W. Everett, was also present:

> It was a Saturday afternoon. The guests were amusing themselves but the host was preparing to slip away. Baden-Powell strolled up beside the waiting motor-car. 'Where are you off to, Pearson?' 'Oh, I am just going over to see a cripple's home. I shan't be long.' The car slid off down the drive, and B-P was left thinking. What he thought was:- 'Here is the man I want to help me – a lover of children, a famous organiser; a great publicity man; he will know how best to start.'[2]

At dinner (by which time Pearson had returned), Baden-Powell spoke about his exploits in South Africa, and of how during the Siege of Mafeking, boys between the ages of twelve and fifteen – whom he had trained – had fulfilled vital roles such as that of postmen, messengers, and stretcher-bearers. He also described the success of his book *Aids to Scouting*. Now, in the early 1900s, Baden-Powell was concerned for Britain's boys, who could easily find themselves at a disadvantage. Those from the working class, because of a lack of education and proper parenting; those from the middle and upper classes, from a lack of self-discipline; and both groups from a lack of moral guidance. He felt that for these reasons they would thus be ill-equipped for the workplace and unlikely to hold down a steady job. He claimed: 'There are one and three-quarter million boys in the country at present, outside the range of good influences, mostly drifting towards hooliganism, for want of a helping hand.'[3]

Baden-Powell outlined how he proposed to utilise his experience of training scouts in the army for the benefit of the youth of Britain, and he declared that Pearson 'was the first public man to whom I spoke of the idea'.[4] Baden-Powell's scheme, said Sidney Dark, captured Pearson's imagination, he was 'immediately attracted to it, by the sport of it, by its open-air atmosphere, and by the fact that it was sure to bring both discipline and interest to growing boys'.[5]

A letter outlining the scheme was sent to prominent and influential figures throughout the country, including members of the Church, State, Army and Navy, in order to enlist their support. This 'met with a most favourable reception'.[6]

It was then a question of finding a suitable name for the proposed new organisation and here, once again, Pearson came to the rescue. He asked Baden-Powell:

> 'What was the name of that book you were telling us about, which you wrote for the Army?' 'Do you mean *Aids to Scouting*?' 'Yes. Why not bring in the word "Scouting"? It has got romance and adventure in it.' Said Baden-Powell, 'You're right. The name "Boy Scout" will appeal, I am sure.' So the Movement became the 'Boy Scout' Movement.[7]

It was also agreed that Baden-Powell would produce a new manual, entitled *Scouting for Boys*.

In 1907, Baden-Powell, urged on by Pearson, devoted himself to working on the text of his new manual, for which he also created the illustrations. They included diagrams of various knots, of the re-setting of a dislocated shoulder, of the lacing-up of a shoe in the scout's way, and of marksmanship. Also included in it was an instruction manual for the benefit of schoolmasters and officers of Boys' and Church Lads' Brigades, and of Cadet Corps.

For Baden-Powell, finding peace in which to work was now essential, and to this end he took up residence in a cottage beneath the windmill on Wimbledon Common. Here, Everett visited him on several occasions, in order to read the proofs of the emerging manuscript. Baden-Powell was ambidextrous and Everett 'was fascinated to watch him writing and sketching, now with his right hand, now with his left'. In February 1908, the manuscript was complete and on 24th of that month Baden-Powell sent it to Pearson.

Between 25 July and 9 August 1907, with the permission of its owner Charles van Raalte, Baden-Powell held an experimental scout camp on Brownsea Island in Poole Harbour, Dorset, where he had sailed with his brothers as a boy. In the spirit of egalitarianism, Baden-Powell invited 20 boys to the camp: ten from public schools; seven from the 1st Bournemouth Boys' Brigade, and three from the 1st Poole Boys' Brigade. Their 'Leaders' included Baden-Powell himself, his nephew and orderly Donald Baden-Powell, a chef, and a coastguard who would give training in first aid.

To this camp, Pearson assigned Percy Everett, who would attend for the final four days in the role of Assistant Scout Master. Said Everett:

> We just imagined a set of boys having a good time on the Island … Well, this is what it was but it was something much more. A trail was being laid at that camp, to be followed by boys and girls, that would reach round the world.[8]

Everett subsequently attended further camps run by Baden-Powell at Humshaugh in Northumberland and at Beaulieu in Hampshire. He became a devoted disciple of Baden-Powell; carrying out scouting exercises, and even tying his shoelaces in the prescribed manner! Everett also had the distinction of being awarded the 6-bead Wood Badge; the only other possessor of that being Baden-Powell himself. Baden-Powell described Everett, who subsequently became the first Deputy Chief Scout, as his 'right hand man'.

This was the origin of the Boy Scout Movement which rapidly spread throughout the world, and in which Pearson had a hand almost from the beginning.

In late 1907 and early 1908, Baden-Powell delivered a series of 50 lectures at various YMCA (Young Men's Christian Association) venues in the larger cities to promote his Boy Scout Movement. Pearson urged that publication of *Scouting for Boys* should be undertaken swiftly, in order to capitalise on the interest which Baden-Powell had generated. The author was quick to agree, stressing in a letter to Pearson's managing director Peter Keary, how important it was 'to catch the public when they are still hot and keen from my lectures'. Before *Scouting for Boys* was published however, there was a degree of editing to be done.

Certain parts of Baden-Powell's original draft of *Scouting for Boys* were not to Pearson's liking and it was either he, or his editor-in-chief Everett, who marked these offending passages in red ink. For example: 'I have told you of the dangers of drink and of smoking which, if indulged in by boys, are certain to make you unhealthy in the end and therefore useless as a scout.' Pearson, however, had no objection to either of these habits, in particular to the latter, as will later be seen. The manuscript continued:

> But there is another practice which [is] perhaps more dangerous than either of them and it is one which is sure to tempt every one of you at one time or another. I speak quite openly. People are much too apt to make it such a secret that many boys never hear the truth and suffer in consequence ... The practice is called 'self-abuse'.

The consequence of such self abuse

> ... is always – mind you *always* – that the boy after a time becomes weak and nervous and shy, he gets headaches and probably palpitations of the heart, and if he still carries it on too far he very often goes out of his mind and becomes an idiot. A very large number of the lunatics in our asylums have made themselves ill by indulging in this vice although at one time they were sensible cheery boys like any one of you.[9]

'Awful diseases' could accrue from such indulgence which could 'rot away the inside of men's mouths, their noses, and eyes, etc.' Baden-Powell then proceeded to give practical advice on how such temptation could be avoided, by the use of cold water and the avoidance of rich food.

This, for Pearson, was too much. He insisted that Baden-Powell omit these paragraphs, and also the excessive and jingoistic references to 'patriotism' and 'imperial decline and fall' which were present under the heading, 'Notes for Instructors'. Baden-Powell's references to 'incontinence' (the absence of self-restraint in respect to sexual desire), were also removed at Pearson's behest, and his references to having a 'daily rear' (meaning, presumably, a bowel evacuation) were substantially reduced.

Pearson assisted Baden-Powell in many ways, by making use of his contacts with the Press to achieve publicity; undertaking the printing of Boy Scout literature; providing the Boy Scout Movement with its first office and a staff of two in London's Henrietta Street. As Baden-Powell had predicted, his movement, energised by Pearson and with the support and expertise of C. Arthur Pearson Ltd became hugely successful.

Scouting for Boys was published, priced fourpence (4d) per issue (each of which was about 70 pages in length) on six alternate Wednesdays, commencing on 15 January 1908. It was produced by Horace Cox, printers to C. Arthur Pearson Ltd. Pearson was heavily involved, both in designing its format and in managing its promotion and marketing. In this, he drew on his previous experience with George Newnes' magazine *Tit-Bits*, and later with his own *Pearson's Weekly*. The front cover of the first number bore the title 'SCOUTING FOR BOYS BY B-P' and a depiction of a boy scout in uniform, looking wistfully out to sea at a ship on the horizon. The message was obvious: for the boy scout, adventure is available to you if you desire it. The inside pages contained an equally winning formula. Here were to be found campfire yarns, written by Baden-Powell himself; extracts from adventure novels (which often contained a bloodthirsty element) such as *Kim* by Rudyard Kipling; a plentiful supply of illustrations; and the promise of more of the same in a fortnight's time. *Scouting for Boys* also told its readers what they must do to become a scout: 'You join a patrol, or … raise a patrol yourself by getting five other boys to join.'

The success of *Scouting for Boys* surprised everybody and when the popular edition was published, it sold at the rate of 5,000 copies per month and was reprinted five times in one year. It eventually became one of the best-selling books of the 20th century, and was translated into numerous languages. For the scouting movement, the outcome was entirely predictable. All over the country, hundreds of scout troops sprung up, both of boys and (perhaps to Baden-Powell's surprise) of girls (The Girl Guide movement was founded in 1910); obliging Baden-Powell to formulate, hastily, the rules and regulations of the movement – which he did almost overnight. On 14 April 1908, the first issue of *The Scout*, a weekly newspaper for boys, was published.

On 26 May 1912, Pearson wrote to Prichard to thank him for arranging cricket coaching for his son Neville, aged 14 and currently a pupil at Eton College. Pearson also appraised Prichard of how matters stood in regard to his failing eyesight. Never one to complain, the former was clearly at a very low ebb indeed:

> I am very much under the weather. The retina of my left eye has split, for some unexplainable reason, and to all intents and purposes depriving that eye of sight, for I only see with it what I can see with my right eye. I have been flat on my back with eyes bandaged for a fortnight now, and have another fortnight of the same joy to look forward to. This is said to be my only chance of saving my sight at all in my left eye, and I want to, as the right one is a very poor creature.[10]

10

Pearson and the National Institute
for the Blind

In 1910, Pearson sold both the *Evening Standard* and the *Standard*, and the following year he relinquished his interest in the *Daily Express*. In 1913, Professor Ernst Fuchs of Vienna informed him that he would soon be blind, and in that year he disposed of his remaining interests in the publishing world.

In October 1913, shortly before his eyesight failed him completely, Pearson joined the Council of the National Institute for the Blind (NIB). He became its treasurer in January 1914, and its first president in July. The NIB had begun life in 1868 as the British and Foreign Society for Improving the Embossed Literature for the Blind. This was based on a system of reading and writing designed for the blind, and invented by French educationist Louis Braille. (In 1953, the NIB became the RNIB – Royal National Institute for the Blind.)

Braille was born in a small town near Paris on 4 January 1809. He was the son of a shoemaker. One day, as a small boy, he entered his father's workshop, picked up an awl (pointed tool used for puncturing holes in leather) and had an accident in which the awl pierced his eye and destroyed the sight in it.

Tragically, some time later, his other eye became infected by the first, and at the age of four he was completely blind.

At the age of ten, Braille was sent to a school for blind boys in Paris, to be taught practical skills, such as applying cane to chairs and making slippers. The boys were also taught to read, by feeling letters which had been embossed on the surface of the page, but not to write. This method was soon to be superseded however. In 1821, a soldier named Charles Barbier visited the school and demonstrated a system which he had invented. It was called 'night writing', and it enabled soldiers to pass instructions along a trench at night, without having to speak, thereby not giving their positions away. It consisted of twelve raised dots which could be arranged to represent different sounds. Braille realised what a valuable tool this was, but not in its present form. He therefore reduced the number of dots to six, and experimented for several years in order to develop the codes necessary for the dots to represent the written word. He also developed similar codes for mathematics and music.

Braille eventually became a teacher at the school at which he had been a student. His system was later adopted throughout the world, but he did not live to see this, for he died of tuberculosis in 1852 at the age of 42.

According to Sidney Dark:

Sir Arthur Pearson ... took a definite and particular interest in the printing and publishing of embossed literature for the blind both in the Braille and Moon types [William Moon, blind inventor and teacher of the blind, who devised a system based on embossed Roman capitals, which is easier to read than Braille, but which occupies more space on the page] with the result that the supply has enormously increased of late years, both in quantity and variety, to the infinite advantage and pleasure of the blind.[1]

Early in 1914, the NIB, which was principally concerned with publishing books in Braille, had moved into new premises in London's Great Portland Street. These were officially opened on 19 March by His Majesty King George V. £30,000 was required to equip the building and in particular to enlarge its library of Braille books and to create an endowment fund for their further manufacture. An account of the occasion reads as follows:

King George, in opening the new premises of the National Institute for the Blind, wished God-speed to the appeal for books in Braille for the sightless, which His Majesty said would, 'break down the barriers shutting out the blind from the common interests of life'.

King George added: 'I am confident your appeal for funds will stir the imagination of many who unreflectingly enjoy the blessings of sight.'[2]

How fortunate for the NIB that they could call on the services of Pearson, for when he joined that organisation its income was a mere £8,000 per annum – barely sufficient to fund its operations. Pearson's skill as a fundraiser was legendary. In the words of St Dunstaner Captain Ian Fraser (later Lord Fraser of Lonsdale, about whom more will be said later): 'Nobody could beat him at getting hard-headed businessmen to dive for their cheque books, or cynical editors and journalists to gobble up blatant puffs and plugs.'[3]

Pearson set about raising the money required in a typically imaginative way: by arranging with the Marconi Telegraph Company for an appeal to be made by their wireless operator at Poldhu, Cornwall to every ship that he could trace that was travelling up and down the English Channel. This, incidentally, was the first time ever that a charitable appeal had been sent out over the airwaves. The appeal stated:

> Books in Braille are practically the only solace of the blind, and, in view of His Majesty's speech, which guarantees the genuineness and urgency of this appeal, may we ask you to arrange during the voyage subscriptions to this first appeal on record made by wireless. The appeal is made to all on board British ships, and even [to] the sympathetic friends on ships flying other flags who are grateful that they are not blind. Kindly send the proceeds to the Lord Mayor's Fund for the Blind, Mansion House, London. This message sent to you gratis by the kindness of the Marconi [Wireless] Company.

At this, one commentator declared enthusiastically:

> The wireless call for help from the sightless will have reached the voyaging millionaire in his thousand guinea suite and the men who do their rough business on the wireless fitted trawlers of the North Sea. The appeal will go on and on, it will be a new Drake's drum beating round the world from the flower-fringed verge of England to the gloomy Magellan Straits, past the corner of the Horn through which Drake himself wound his way to the conquest of the Spanish Main. It will raise the drowsy languor of a trooper in the Red Sea and startle the pearl fishers of the Pacific. The outward bound emigrant, with all his life before him, will hear of it in common with the colonial going home with all his life behind him. It will echo up the

Adriatic and drift to the sealers lying fearfully at anchor in the white fog of the frozen north. It is a great appeal sent forth in a great way.[4]

Pearson also persuaded the Lord Mayor of London to open the Mansion House Fund, to which he, along with Lord Northcliffe and Lord Rothermere, each contributed the sum of £1,000 from their own pockets. He also persuaded the Archbishops of Canterbury and Westminster, together with the leaders of the Free Churches, to hold a special service of thanksgiving for the blessing of sight; with the result that over 40,000 such services were held simultaneously throughout the country and a great deal more money was raised.

Pearson, it will be remembered, had given Baden-Powell considerable assistance in launching his Scout Movement. Now it was time for the favour to be repaid. Pearson wrote to Hadyn Dimmock who worked for *The Scout* magazine, to see if he could think of a way of involving the scouts in fund-raising for the NIB's appeal, bearing in mind that it was contrary to the principles of the Scout Movement to beg or to collect money. The outcome was that at Dimmock's suggestion, on 2 May 1914 Baden-Powell made the request that 'All scouts perform a "good turn" for *The Scout* magazine publisher Mr C. Arthur Pearson, in order to raise money for his scheme of publishing literature in Braille for the blind.' Within a year, the sum of £60,000 had been raised and by 1921, the NIB's annual income had risen to £358,174.[5]

Pearson stated that it was shortly before the start of the First World War in 1914, that his eyes failed him completely.[6] So, how did he face up to the reality of blindness? The answer is summed up succinctly by C. B. Fry, who described him as 'the man who … went blind with such wonderful courage … and who never gave in to his disability'.[7]

When war broke out in August 1914, the Prince of Wales asked Pearson to be director of the National Relief Fund, one of the aims of which was to alleviate distress amongst demobilised service personnel. The outcome was that Pearson became Joint Honorary Secretary of that organisation's Collecting Committee, and in less than six months, raised the sum of £1,000,000.

11

Pearson and the Founding
of St Dunstan's

On 4 August 1914, Great Britain declared war on Germany. In that year, the Pearsons sold Frensham Place and relocated to Bourne End in Hertfordshire. Because of its stables and indoor riding school, the property was now requisitioned by the military for use as a training centre for recruits to the cavalry.

A blinded Belgian soldier was in an English hospital in 1914 and Pearson went to see him several times. Soon after, Pearson learned of two English soldiers who had lost their sight: a sergeant and a private, both of whom had been taken to the 2nd London General Hospital, Chelsea (which before the war had been St Mark's College) and he promptly went to see them also. From then on, said Pearson:

At least once a week it was my practice to visit the hospital, to see especially the men who had newly arrived. I felt that because I too was blind I might speak to these men of their future more convincingly than if I had not shared the same experience and faced the same problems.[1]

Pearson now had a vision of creating an establishment, especially dedicated to caring for blinded soldiers and sailors:

> The main idea that animated me in establishing this Hostel for the blinded
> soldiers was that the sightless men, after being discharged from hospital, might
> come into a little world where the things which blind men cannot do, were
> forgotten and where everyone was concerned with what blind men can do.
>
> They would naturally need to be looked after and to be trained, and I was
> convinced that their future happiness, their success, everything, in short,
> would depend on the atmosphere with which they were surrounded.[2]

The question was where were the blinded soldiers to be trained when they
left hospital? In the event, it was a German banker and patron of the arts,
Otto Kahn, who came to the rescue. Otto Hermann Kahn was born in
Mannheim, Germany in 1867. Having trained as a banker, he worked in
London before moving to New York City in 1893. Here, he joined Kuhn,
Loeb & Co., a firm of investment bankers. Kahn, however, was in two minds
about whether or not to return to England.

Canadian-born British newspaper magnate and politician Max Aitken
(later Lord Beaverbrook) suggested to Kahn that if he wished to be accepted
into the life of the City of London, there were two things which it would
be advisable for him to do. The first was to stand for Parliament. The second
was to purchase Pearson's *Daily Express* newspaper, which was running into
financial difficulties. This is how Kahn and Pearson met.

In fact, although Kahn went as far as to offer the sum of £30,000 for the
Daily Express, he had second thoughts both about this venture and about a
career in politics. He therefore decided to remain in the USA. Nevertheless,
he retained his home, 'St Dunstan's Lodge' in London's Regent's Park, which
he had rented from Henry Hucks Gibbs (First Lord Altringham) since 1912.
This was a large mansion, built at the time of the Regency (1810–1820),
designed by the famous architect Decimus Burton and was once owned by
the third Marquess of Hertford.

Having heard in 1914 that Pearson was looking for premises for his
blinded men, Kahn generously placed St Dunstan's Lodge at his disposal.
As Dark declared: 'St Dunstan's has all the advantages of a large country
house with a wonderful garden, though it is within a couple of miles of
Central London's Piccadilly Circus.' The garden was 15 acres in size, and
second only to that of Buckingham Palace. It included a lake contiguous
with the larger one in nearby Regent's Park.

Before the blinded soldiers could move into St Dunstan's Lodge it was
necessary to make some alterations to the building. It was now that a Mrs

Lewis Hall, described by Pearson as 'a continuous benefactor to the blinded men', came to the rescue by lending him a house at 6 Bayswater Hill, which would be known as The Blinded Soldiers and Sailors Hostel. It was opened in early February 1915 with two blinded soldiers in residence.

In order that no war-blinded serviceman should be overlooked, it was necessary for Pearson to enlist the cooperation of Surgeon-General Sir Alfred Keogh. This he did, and thereafter, 'every effort was made to send all the blinded men [soldiers and sailors] when they reached England to the 2nd London General Hospital.'[3] Here, Pearson would talk to them about what the organisation could offer them and explain what type of training could be given. The result was that 'With practically no exceptions all the soldiers and sailors of the British Imperial Forces blinded in the war came under my care, in order that they might learn to be blind.'[4] The expression, 'learning to be blind' was a favourite one of Pearson's.

The temporary hostel in Bayswater was staffed by a matron, male orderlies, and a small number of Voluntary Aid Detachment nurses ('VADs', created by the Red Cross prior to the First World War). The VADs would also act as cooks, kitchen maids, and laundresses.

Finally, on 26 March 1915 the hostel relocated from Bayswater to its new premises in Regent's Park, where in the large conservatory, various handicrafts were taught. By this time the number of St Dunstaners had risen to sixteen. Pearson was delighted, for this was the perfect place for his men to be rehabilitated: 'No sound is [heard] here of the London traffic ... The rustle of the breeze in the foliage is creative to the blind man – making the trees stand out clearly to his mental vision.'[5]

In addition to providing training to blinded servicemen from Britain and the Empire, according to Pearson,

> We also had the pleasure of welcoming one French officer and three French private soldiers whom I had met while on a visit to the various establishments throughout France at which French blinded soldiers were cared for, and who had evinced a particular desire to make a stay with us.

Soon, St Dunstan's was bursting at the seams!

The problem of overcrowding was alleviated, to some degree, when Sir John and Lady Stirling-Maxwell lent their house, a mile or so away at 21 Portland Place, for St Dunstan's blinded officers. This is also where

Pearson lived, except during the holidays when he returned to his home at Bourne End. All too soon, even the Stirling-Maxwell's house, large as it was, proved to be inadequate for the purpose. So another house, almost exactly opposite to it in Portland Place was rented, together with several flats in the neighbourhood, which were placed at the disposal of married officers. Pearson was adamant, however, that in their training at St Dunstan's, officers and other ranks were to be treated exactly alike.

Not only had the owner of St Dunstan's, Otto Kahn, placed his house at the service of the blinded service personnel completely free of all charges, including the cost of maintenance of the grounds, and to some extent of the house itself, but he was also a generous benefactor of the hostel's general funds.

St Dunstan's came to acquire its name through a complex chain of circumstances. In London's Fleet Street stands the Church of St Dunstan-in-the-West. This church possessed a clock, built by Thomas Harrys in 1671, which was attached to the side of the building. The clock, which was of a substantial size, was unique in that it was the first one ever to be made which displayed the minutes as well as the hours. When the church was refurbished, funds were needed, so the decision was made to sell the clock. It was then purchased by the third Marquess of Hertford (for the sum of 200 guineas) who set it up in the grounds of his London residence. A feature of the clock was two giant figures, carved in oak, who struck the hours and the quarter hours upon an anvil. The Marquess was particularly fond of it because as a child his nanny would take him to see the giants strike the bell as a treat whenever he had been well behaved. It was famously mentioned in several works of English literature, including: *Fortunes of Nigel* by Sir Walter Scott; *A Tale of Two Cities* by Charles Dickens; *The Warden* by Anthony Trollope; and in several poems by William Cowper. Having purchased this magnificent clock, the Marquess renamed his dwelling St Dunstan's Villa.[6] (The clock was returned to the church in Fleet Street in 1935.)

Pearson believed, erroneously, that St Dunstan was the patron saint of the blind. However, Dunstan was generally regarded, since the Middle Ages, as the patron saint of goldsmiths and silversmiths and is most frequently represented holding a pair of smith's tongs. He was born in Glastonbury, Somerset in 924, where a church had been founded in the first century by St Joseph of Arimathea (a disciple of Jesus Christ) who had brought with him the Holy Grail. This church became Glastonbury Abbey, built by the Benedictine order of monks in the tenth to eleventh centuries.

Having been educated at Glastonbury Abbey, Dunstan took monastic vows. In 945, he was appointed Abbot of Glastonbury by King Edmund and he set about renovating the abbey and establishing it as a centre of religious teaching. Dunstan went on to become Bishop of Worcester, then of London and finally, in 961, Archbishop of Canterbury. His Feast Day is 19 May.

The question now arises, who is the patron saint of the blind? About this, there is considerable difference of opinion amongst the various branches of the Christian Church. In fact, amongst the dozen or so contenders for this honour are St Odelia (French, 7th century); St Lucy (Santa Lucia, Sicilian, 3rd century); St Raphael the Archangel; St Alice (Belgian, 13th century); and the twin brothers St Cosmos and St Damien (Syrian, 4th century).

12

The Newcomer to St Dunstan's

One may picture a visit by Pearson (or a member of his staff) to the hospital bedside of a newly-blinded soldier, who is likely be experiencing emotions such as grief, rage and bitterness. Pearson places his cards on the table and offers the man a place at his hostel. He is met with scepticism, but he persists. After all, he has done this many times before. Not only that, but Pearson, as has already been demonstrated, is something of an (amateur) authority on the human mind, having written a number of books on how to gain an insight into a person's character.

Pearson explains about St Dunstan's in particular that it is not a home where people are to be shut away for the rest of their lives. Neither is it simply an institution. On the contrary, training is offered, which will enable those who wish to do so, to learn a trade and thereby regain their independence so that they can support their family and become a useful member of society.

Finally, Pearson, never one to beat about the bush but also with some sense of of the dramatic, reveals that he himself is blind.

The man considers the alternatives. Almost invariably, he realises that there are none. And there is something about this stranger that he feels he can trust. Yet there must still be some terrible doubt at the back of his mind, the feeling that he is beyond help.

Before Pearson leaves the man's bedside there is a ritual to be performed: a seemingly small affair, but one of symbolic weight. He presents the man with a Braille watch. After explaining briefly about the raised dots which replace the numbers, and how to open it with the winder in a certain position, he lets the man explore the watch. Pearson reassures him by saying that it is really quite easy to use, and he will get used to it very quickly. He tells the man that this is his first step to independence; now he can tell the time.

Once the blinded man has accepted the invitation to St Dunstan's, things swing into action. Before he has even left hospital, arrangements are made for him to receive regular visits from a lady tutor (one of dozens who have been recruited by St Dunstan's from the staff of the National Library for the Blind), who gives him a daily lesson in Braille. Other staff would teach him to use a typewriter and how to make string bags. The men also had their letters read to them, and were helped to write their own. Newsworthy topics of the day were discussed, in order to keep their minds occupied and to prevent them from becoming bored. This is an essential prelude to the man's rehabilitation, for as St Dunstan's Consultant Ophthalmologist Sir Arnold Lawson pointed out:

> The sudden plunging of the sighted man into darkness by the havoc of a shell-burst or bullet, must be, and is, followed by a period of mental depression often of the most acute character, which persists in many persons for long periods.[1]

It is, therefore, essential to make every effort to prevent this happening.

On release from hospital, the blinded soldier is taken across London, by taxi, to St Dunstan's, Regent's Park. Here, he is greeted in the traditional manner by a cadre of Boy Scouts who take care of his luggage, pay his taxi fare, and introduce him to a VAD whose task it is to sit in the hallway and register new arrivals.

He then reports to Matron, who allocates him a bed in a dormitory; shows him where to put his clothes, and reads him the house rules. She introduces him to the Dispensary Nurse, who will give him all the necessary attention in respect of his injuries, and then to some of the blind residents who are sitting in comfort in the lounge. Finally, she offers him a meal.

Pearson realised that if he was to have any chance of success with his blinded men, it was first necessary to gain their trust. To this end, on the day following his admission to St Dunstan's, the newcomer would receive an invitation from the 'Chief' to see him in his private office at 12 noon. Shortly afterwards, his relatives would also be interviewed.

Had he been able to do so, the man would have observed a dapper-looking gentleman with receding, grey hair, in a single-breasted suit (with waistcoat), tie, and black, shiny shoes. The newcomer, however, is aware only of Pearson's voice. Journalist and author Richard King Huskinson, described by Pearson as 'one of our most devoted helpers', sets the scene:

A guide leads in the blinded soldier and he finds Sir Arthur standing to welcome him; somehow or other, the hands of the two blind men meet. Sitting on the sofa, still holding the hand of his visitor, Sir Arthur begins at once to talk of the future.

No one can understand the power that one man has over another. If you were present at one of these interviews; if you attempted to analyse Sir Arthur's secret, you would probably say that he took it for granted that the blinded man was going to make a success of being blind. In a word, the man finds himself swept along by Sir Arthur's unfaltering convictions ... And you see the change in the man taking place, you hear a new tone in his voice – he has been carried over the dead point, and you realise that there will be no going back in his mind.

As for sympathy, it has been expressed by the touch of the hand resting on his, by Sir Arthur's genuine interest in his affairs. Eyes are not needed to catch the deep feeling under the brisk, confident tone in which everything has been said. The man knows that all is understood – this, more than anything else, makes a cheerful discussion of the future assuring. The sense of assurance is what, above all, is requisite. He finds himself laughing at difficulties, in better spirits, one would judge, than he had experienced since he was wounded. These interviews do not last very long, but they are very momentous, and he is an exceptional man who does not leave the room merely with a determination to make a success of his life, but with a new-found confidence that he can do so.[2]

For the newcomer to St Dunstan's there were huge practical difficulties to surmount, not least that of being able to find his way about. As far as moving from room to room was concerned, St Dunstan's had an ingenious system whereby 'pathways' of linoleum ran through the fitted carpets. A man could, therefore, feel the change of floor covering when he walked on it, and was thereby able to find his way around. Also, the edge of the carpet was easily detectable with the aid of the stout walking stick (which each man had been issued – white sticks having not yet come into use). Generally however, St Dunstaners managed without the aid of sticks, as Pearson himself proudly acknowledged.

As they walk along, said Pearson, some of the men 'sing out in a cheery voice to clear a way for themselves'.[3] In any event, there was no doubt in his mind who was to have priority on the 'pathways':

> Visitors are requested not to stand about on the linoleum paths, or even to walk on them. They are solely for the use of the blind men who hear one another coming and going and after a few weeks – in some cases a very few days – walk about the great house with a firmness and readiness which leads many people to find it very difficult indeed to believe that they cannot see where they are going.

Likewise, the tops and bottoms of staircases were indicated by patches of rubber or wood, which the feet could instantly detect. Also, etched into the banisters were numbered notches, each corresponding with a particular step. In this way, having been told how many steps there were in total, the man would be able to work out how many there were to go before he reached the top or bottom. Outside, there were ropes and handrails to guide him, with bosses set on top of their supporting wooden posts, to signify junctions. These posts were padded with straw wound around with felt, so that the men would not injure themselves, should they happen to bump against them.

There were many other little tricks to be learned that would make life easier. For example, by cupping of a finger over the lip of a glass, over-pouring could be avoided; and lining up a cigarette end with the end of the match before striking, ensured that the flame was in exactly the correct position to ignite the tip.

For those who wished to go walking, rowing on the nearby Regent's Park Lake, or to take part in in physical drill, their day would begin at 6.30 a.m. Drill was usually conducted by a sighted, ex-army, non-commissioned officer, and occasionally by a St Dunstaner who could detect by ear when a man was not keeping good time with the others! Officially, however, the day commenced with breakfast at 8 a.m., after which the newspaper was read out by a sighted person. This included news from the Front, which of pourse being of particular interest, was read at length.[4]

Letters were delivered and read to the men by the VAD staff – described by Fraser as 'wonderfully charming and attentive'.[5] The VADs became the blind men's companions. They were able to describe to them what the various members of staff looked like.

At 9.30 a.m. a whistle was blown for work to commence. From 12 a.m. the men were free to relax in the lounge, take a walk, or write letters until 1 p.m., when a bell was rung to signal lunchtime. At 2.30 p.m. the whistle was blown again and work recommenced until 4.30 p.m. From this time, the men were left to their own devices. After supper, taken at 8 p.m., there were newspaper readings for those who wished to attend. Alternatively, a person might prefer to hear a story read to him by one of the nursing staff. Finally, at 9.30 p.m. an orderly conducted the men to their various dormitories, and by 10 p.m., everyone was expected to be in bed.

Sometimes, whilst promenading in the garden, the men would encounter Ruby Smith, born at St Dunstan's Lodge in 1912. She was the 4-year-old daughter of the Head Gardener. Ruby brought a new dimension to the lives of the blind men, reminding them of their own childhood and those that had them of their own children. Ruby recalled:

> I used to go up to them and chat, and we'd walk around just holding hands … I used to ask them where they wanted to go. If they wanted to go to a certain workshop, I knew them all by heart. I knew where to find everything and I just used to paddle along with them. They were so pleased to have a child come and talk to them. I always remember how my little hand seemed so small in theirs.[6]

Ruby's weekly task was to bring the Chief a bouquet of roses, picked by her father.

13

Types of Eye Injury Sustained and Treatment

Pearson was unstinting in his praise for, and gratitude to, 'the distinguished specialists in almost every branch of the medical profession, who freely placed their invaluable services at our disposal.'[1] They included the 'eminent voluntary oculists and the doctor', who visited daily to attend to the men's eyes, and also to those on the sick list and to those who had become more seriously ill and 'were cared for in our own little private hospital'.

The 'eminent oculists' referred to, were Sir Arnold Lawson, who was Senior Ophthalmic Surgeon and Lecturer in Ophthalmic Surgery at London's Middlesex Hospital, and Brevet-Major Arthur William Ormond of the Royal Army Medical Corps, Ophthalmic Surgeon at the 2nd London General Hospital, Chelsea and also at London's Guy's Hospital. During the wartime period, a total of 825 men came under Lawson's care, as compared with 1,008 for Ormond.

Lawson had promised (in 1920) that he would write a book, an account of the medical (ophthalmic) work which he performed from 1915–1920. Entitled *War Blindness at St Dunstan's*, and published in 1922, it includes details of how the men lost their sight.

As for Pearson, Lawson describes the Chief in his book as, 'a man blinded at middle age, endowed with great intellectual capacity and marvellous powers of organisation.' Pearson's greatest achievement, he said, was to realise 'that it was still possible for him to carry on after his loss [of sight] as well and in some ways better than he had done before'.[2]

A study of *War Blindness at St Dunstan's* leads to a remarkable conclusion: that 417 out of the 825 of Lawson's patients, had lost their sight for reasons *other than* those directly connected with their wartime service – in other words, through accident and disease. Of these 417 cases of so-called 'Non-traumatic Blindness', no less than 127 had lost their sight through being infected with the venereal disease syphilis, which has the capacity to damage not only the eye, but also the optic nerve and even the brain itself. In fact, 33 of these men were suffering from *tabes dorsalis* – an advanced stage of syphilis in which the spinal cord is affected. Another appalling legacy of syphilis is that, in its final stages, it renders the sufferer insane; it was for this reason that many St Dunstaners ended their days in psychiatric hospitals. At the other end of the spectrum, Lawson cites the cases of five St Dunstaner 'lads' aged 20, 21, 22, 22, and 25 respectively, all of whom were already quite blind from syphilitic infection. So how had they become infected? Clearly these men, many of whom were away from their homes and families, wives and girl friends for the very first time, had sought solace in the arms of Belgian and French prostitutes. Sadly, in those days, no antibiotics were available with which to treat them.

Other causes of blindness in this category were the presence of a tumour within the brain, and cerebro-spinal meningitis. There were also eleven cases of glaucoma – the very same disease which had caused Pearson himself to become blind.

Those whose blindness was directly attributable to traumatic injuries – the so-called 'Traumatic Blindness' category – numbered 407, and Lawson again subdivided these according to cause. (Here, it should be remembered that for a person to be able to see, the whole of the visual pathway – from the retina of the eye to the visual cortex, and from there to regions of the brain which are concerned with interpretation of shapes, moving objects and so forth – must be intact.)

Seventy-two cases had suffered bullet wounds of the orbits (the bony hollows in which the eyeballs rest) often as the result of a man going 'over the top', or as a victim of enemy snipers. The Belgian, whom Pearson had visited in hospital in 1914, had lost his sight in this way. So had Ian Fraser, who not only became a St Dunstaner, but also played a significant part in the development of that organisation, as will shortly be seen.

Included in Lawson's 'Traumatic Blindness' group were seventeen men whose blindness was caused by fractures of the back (occipital region) of the skull. The occipital lobes – one on each side of the rear part of the brain – contain the main centre for the processing of visual information, the so-called visual cortex, damage to which may result in blindness. Another twelve men had been blinded on account of fractures of bones adjacent to the apex (rear) of the orbits and the optic canals (through which the optic nerves travel). Sixteen of the men had experienced concussion from the explosion of a shell or bomb. In these cases the blast alone had been of such severity as to cause damage to the brain and, in particular, to the visual cortex, which had rendered them permanently blind.

Of the 289 'Miscellaneous Cases' in the 'Traumatic Blindness' category, all had been blinded by 'direct smashing injuries from in front, or by perforation of the globes [eyeballs] by fragments of metal or other flying bodies'.[3] In only two of these cases was blindness caused by bayonet wounds.

A number of these St Dunstaners had been blinded in the most extraordinary circumstances. One was using a detonator as a pencil case, believing it to be empty. When he rammed a pencil into it with particular force, it exploded, blinding him in both eyes. Another was using a 16-inch metal file as a cricket bat when it flew out of its handle, perforating his left eye and fracturing the right orbit. The right eye had to be removed and the left remained permanently blind through damage to the tissues behind the eyeball.

In another case, when a company had taken over a building from the enemy, a man was ordered by his sergeant to chop up some wood which was lying in a corner. As he was chopping, the wood exploded. The timber had apparently been hollowed out and an egg-bomb placed inside. (This event had occurred only two days before the signing of the Armistice.) A man tripped when attempting to force his way through a barbed-wire entanglement. In his fall, his left eye was pierced by the barbed wire, which also damaged the cornea of his right eye. The left eye had to be removed.

The 19-year-old pilot of a wartime aircraft collided with another aircraft whilst taxiing and experienced a severe blow to the upper part of his face. Although the eyes showed no signs of external injury, both retinas were severely damaged. Another pilot was shot down, whereupon his aircraft caught fire. Although he was extricated from it, he was 'horribly burnt all over his face, arms, and body'. As for his eyes, there was very severe corneal ulceration which almost destroyed the sight in one eye. In the other, there was 'a large, bulging corneal scar with adherent iris' and raised intra-ocular pressure. Lawson, therefore, performed an iridectomy (surgical removal of part of the iris) which successfully reduced the pressure and enabled the man to retain sufficient sight for him 'to see about the room and recognise large objects fairly close to him'. Sadly, he died a year or so later.[4]

Gas and Blindness

Gas weapons were used for the first time in August 1914 by the French, in the form of tear-gas grenades containing xylyl bromide. This was contrary to the terms of the Hague Convention, which forbade the use of 'poison or poisoned weapons'.[5] This substance is an irritant rather than a gas that can kill. The low concentrations had a negligible effect.

The first major use of poison gas was at the commencement of the second Battle of Ypres on 22 April 1915, when the German Pioneer Regiment No.35 employed chlorine gas against French positions near Boezinge, situated to the north of Ypres in the Ypres Salient. As its density is approximately 2.5 times greater than that of air, chlorine gas, when released, will initially remain close to the ground, provided that there is little air movement. It is, therefore, an ideal substance to be floated across no man's land to the enemy trench, into which it will sink.

The men had no gas masks (the 'box respirator' – where a mask was attached by a separate pipe to a filter – was not issued until late in 1916). The only counter-measure was for the soldier to soak his handkerchief or puttees in water or urine, and clap it over his face – something which there was hardly the time or the opportunity to do in the heat of battle. Eyes are seldom damaged severely by chlorine gas, although temporary blindness may result. However, burns to the cornea may lead to corneal ulceration, and subsequent scarring.

The Germans went on to produce more lethal varieties of gas, including phosgene in December 1915, and mustard gas in mid-1917. Phosgene is a highly toxic, irritating and corrosive gas. If it comes into contact with the eye, it reacts slowly with moisture therein to produce hydrochloric acid. Mustard gas (so-called because of its aroma) has the ability to penetrate clothing and all types of gas mask that were then in service. It causes irritation of the eyes, swelling of the eyelids and sensitivity to light. Vision is lost as the corneas become ulcerated and then decay. It also causes blisters to form on the skin, which may turn gangrenous.

A harrowing image of the First World War is that of soldiers who have been the victims of a gas attack. They walk slowly in procession, each with a hand on the shoulder of the one in front, as they are guided by a sighted person to the regimental first-aid post. This scene was immortalised by John Singer Sargent in his painting 'Gassed'.

In view of the widespread use of increasingly toxic forms of poison gas in the First World War, it might be supposed that St Dunstan's would be inundated with the victims of gas attacks. This was not the case, although several men whose eyes had been damaged by gas were admitted during the period of hostilities. The reason for this was that usually, if the damage was severe enough to blind, then it was severe enough to kill, due to damage to the lungs from the effects of inhalation. However, for those that did survive a gas attack, the symptoms of it might not appear until years later.

The Saint Dunstan's Annual, published in 1935, contained a disturbing article, stating that even seventeen years after the end of the First World War, men continued to lose their sight as a result of the gas poisoning which they had received in 1917 or 1918. They included five new cases in the previous twelve months alone. There was no doubt that the culprit was not lachrymatory gases (such as tear gas) or chlorine, but mustard gas.[6]

Treatment

In respect of injuries to the eyes, although urgent medical treatment, including surgery, was given both in the theatre of war and in dedicated UK hospitals, such as the London General Hospital, Chelsea, there were several conditions which presented ongoing problems.

Interstitial keratitis is a condition in which blood vessels grow into the cornea and render it opaque. It may be the result of a traumatic injury to the cornea, or of an infection such as syphilis. It was treated by iridectomy, which was believed to improve the nutrition of the eye. Detachment of the retina was treated by scleral trephining, whereby a small incision was made into the white of the eye (sclera) in order to reduce the pressure within. Glaucoma was also treated by scleral trephining and iridectomy; the object again being to reduce the pressure in the eyes which would otherwise destroy the optic nerve. (This was the same operation which Pearson himself had undergone, but without success.)

In mild cases of traumatic cataract (opacity of the lens due to trauma), a 'cataract lens' (magnifying glass) was prescribed to improve the vision. However, if the cataract was so dense that it seriously impeded the vision, then, with the patient's consent, it was surgically removed. Inflamed, or discharging eyes and eye sockets, required frequent bathing and irrigation at one of St Dunstan's two dispensaries.

Although a number of St Dunstaners possessed corneas that Lawson described as hazy, he makes no mention of having performed a corneal graft. Evidently, this was not common practice in those days; even though the first corneal graft was performed as early as 1905 by the Viennese ophthalmologist Eduard Zirm.

Artificial, or 'glass' eyes were offered to fill empty sockets. However, those men who disliked the idea of wearing one were at liberty to request that Lawson close the lids permanently with sutures.

Some men, who were only temporarily blinded, joined St Dunstan's briefly but left when their sight returned. Sadly, however, despite the best efforts of the medical profession, it proved impossible to save the sight of the vast majority of the men who were admitted to St Dunstan's between 1914 and 1918. The same was true of the majority of those who were admitted subsequently, suffering from the long-term effects of their injuries or illnesses. For as Lawson said: 'No matter how quiet the eyes, or how long a time the disease has been stationary, old inflammatory mischief is always apt to recrudesce under conditions inimical to general health.'[7]

In some cases a degree of improvement was obtained, and in any event, it was of some comfort to the men to know that they were being attended to on an ongoing basis by two of the finest ophthalmologists in London. It should also be mentioned that in addition to the medical and ophthalmic specialists, there was a 'great army of men and women' who helped Pearson in his work, 'the majority of them giving up their time without any payment'.[8]

14

Pearson's Brainchild in Operation

Medical Care

The most seriously injured of those admitted to St Dunstans were sent to the Torquay Annexe for convalescence. Its staff included a medical officer and doctor, a matron, a fully-trained nursing staff and a chaplain. Alternatively, those who required operative treatment might be sent to St Dunstan's Hospital in Sussex Place, London, or to one of the London hospitals. If required, St Dunstan's would then arrange for a period of convalescence at one of its annexes.

For the amputee, artificial limbs were provided, and in the case of those who had lost one or both arms, a series of experiments began to discover which type of prosthesis was best suited to the patient's needs. Every effort was made to accommodate such men, even to the extent of races being organised for one-armed oarsmen on nearby Regent's Park Lake.

Work

Pearson 'very quickly … realised that it is the blind man who, above all, needs occupation, and that the more active, the more normal he can make his life, the happier he will be.'[1] He acknowledged, however, that some men were unable to work, either because of severe physical injury, or mental trauma. In this case, St Dunstan's would provide accommodation for them at one of its convalescent annexes. St Dunstaner Ian Fraser happily said that there were very few such men because Pearson 'succeeded in inspiring almost anyone who could work, with the desire *to* work'.[2]

Having worked for the NIB, Pearson was highly enthusiastic about Braille, and the aim was to teach this skill to as many St Dunstaners as possible – it would clearly be impossible for those who had lost hands, or whose hands were seriously injured. Whilst he acknowledged that Braille was a difficult skill to learn, Pearson declared that there was

> … a special delight in [a man] being able to read to himself, above all because in this way is provided a resource which enables him to fill in any unoccupied time when he happens to be alone. It gives him entrance to the world of books and brings back to him some of the independence he has lost.
>
> Not only books, but monthly magazines and weekly newspapers are produced in Braille – and between blind people correspondence by this medium is carried on without the need of relying on a sighted person to read aloud the letters received.
>
> To be able to write in Braille is a great advantage in that it enables a blind man to record and read his own notes and attend personally to his private business papers. Many of the soldiers who are now poultry-farmers and tradesmen keep their accounts in Braille with complete success.[3]

As an incentive, every man who passed the Braille reading test was, on leaving St Dunstan's, presented with a Braille writing machine. Furthermore, to those who passed the Braille writing test, which was much more difficult, Pearson gave a gold watch-chain.[4]

The men were also taught to type, and when they had passed the typewriting test, each was presented with a Remington typewriter. Shorthand typing was also taught, the words being taken down on a small machine through which a thin paper ribbon passed, and on which the signs denoting the various words and phrases were embossed.[5] Telephony was a popular subject, and more than 100 St Dunstaners became telephonists – many going on to spend their entire career with one company.[6]

Massage (or physiotherapy, as it is called today) was also popular and there was a great demand by hospitals all over the country for qualified masseurs.

The preliminary course of massage instruction offered by St Dunstan's provided excellent opportunities for jokes and pranks, as, for example, when a trainee masseur placed a skeleton, used to demonstrate practical anatomy – complete with bowler hat, scarf and pipe – at the front door of the physiotherapy classroom. This was just before the Chief was due to arrive to show a distinguished visitor around! After completing a preliminary course a trainee would then undergo an advanced training course at the National Institute for the Blind in Great Portland Street, London, at the end of which he sat the examination of the Incorporated Society of Trained Masseurs.

Poultry farming was popular with St Dunstaners – both from Britain and from the Empire – some of whom had worked on farms before they were blinded. Their mentor was Captain F. Pierson-Webber, a former soldier who had been blinded by the sun whilst serving in Africa. He taught the men to rear chickens with the aid of an incubator. Pearson said: 'It is a remarkable sight to watch the blind men handling the chickens, distinguishing the different breeds by the sense of touch, judging the quality of eggs, selecting the different foodstuffs.'[7]

The most popular of all the trades taught at St Dunstan's was boot-repairing or 'snobbing', as the men nicknamed it. The course, which normally lasted for 8 months (other courses lasted longer), was combined with mat making, and for a very good reason: for as Pearson said, when the men found themselves out in the workplace, the work was likely to be intermittent: 'There may be twenty pairs of boots to repair one week and only half a dozen the next. In a slack week the man can make a few mats and have the advantage of a change of work.'[8]

Pearson describes a typical scene in the workshop:

A very large number of men are busy here – it is a scene of intense, orderly activity and movement; and on all sides you will hear men whistling or singing as they work. The Cobblers' Chorus, accompanied by blows of hammer upon leather sole, is a never-ending source of wonder and delight to the visitor.[9]

He went on to say how careful the novice boot-repairer was to affix his first sole to the shell of the boot, and then shape and finish it, using leather of the best quality supplied to them by St Dunstan's, and how the skilled instructor 'permitted nothing to pass that was not first-rate'.[10] Visitors to St Dunstan's were fascinated to watch, as the men put a handful of tingles (fine nails) into their mouths, then push them forward one at a time and hold them between their lips, ready to be taken and used. There was an ingeniously designed punch by which holes could be made, at intervals, around the perimeter of the sole. Then, all the blind man had to do was to feel for these holes to determine exactly where each tingle should go.

When they had achieved a degree of proficiency, the men were entrusted to repair the footwear of the local people of St John's Wood, who were only too willing to show an interest and support the cause. Also, four or five pairs of army boots per week were taken in to be repaired.

Carpentry and joinery were enjoyed so much by the men that according to Fraser, few of them downed tools when the whistle blew at 4.30 p.m. and sometimes carried on with their making of cabinets, picture frames, dog kennels etc. until well into the evening, when 'visitors were sometimes startled to hear the sounds of hammering and sawing executed with confidence [yet] coming from a completely dark workshop.'[11]

As a less 'industrial' output, St Dunstan's was famous for its production of string bags, which were knitted on a traditional, circular, wooden frame, with pegs spaced at 1-inch intervals around its perimeter. Two lengths of string were then pleated to make the handles. There was friendly rivalry amongst the men as to who could knit a string bag the quickest, and when a man broke the record, he earned the nickname 'The Bag King'! Netting for tennis nets, hammocks, and fruit cages was also made.

Motivation

Consultant Ophthalmologist Sir Arnold Lawson, stated that in respect of work, motivating the blinded officers sometimes proved more difficult than motivating the other ranks. This was because the officers were, more often than not, in receipt of comparatively larger incomes, and therefore had less incentive to work. The non-commissioned men, on the other hand, were obliged to augment their pensions by any means in their power.[12]

Nevertheless, many of the officers did achieve success: Captain Angus Buchanan, for example, the only holder of the Victoria Cross to be blinded in the First World War. Prior to enlisting in the army Buchanan had been an undergraduate at Oxford University reading law. Having completed his period at St Dunstan's, he returned to the university in 1919, graduated, became articled to a firm of solicitors and finally went into partnership with a legal practice in Gloucestershire.[13] F. le Gros Clark became a writer of short stories, children's stories and novels. He later developed an interest in health and nutrition, and worked for the United Nations Food and Agriculture Organisation. Of the other St Dunstaner officers, one was able to return to work as a chartered accountant, another as a solicitor, a third as a barrister and several more as company directors. Fraser, however, issued a caveat. There were some men who even St Dunstan's, with all the expertise and enthusiasm of its staff, could not succeed in motivating.

Leisure

It was generally acknowledged that the men of St Dunstan's learned at a faster rate than those at other institutions for the blind; the reason being, said Pearson, that 'the men are put to play before they can feel brain-fag and mental strain.'[14] One of Pearson's own recreations was to gallop his horse 'fearlessly over the Downs', even when he had lost his sight completely, and he certainly appreciated the importance of leisure.[15] In accordance with this philosophy, he introduced a number of activities into the curriculum

> ... which were designed, not merely to bring gaiety to the lives of the blinded men, but to draw out their powers of enjoyment. To instruct them in practical accomplishments was a very important part of our work, but it was not everything. My plan went far beyond that. Indeed it seemed to me that the blinded man required more encouragement in the direction of play than in that of work.[16]

Outdoor pastimes were encouraged, such as tandem-cycling, swimming, walking and running races, and physical drill. Boxing and wrestling matches were held regularly in the gymnasium. Pearson enthused about how the men took to rowing on nearby Regent's Park Lake:

> To the blinded, man there is joy in being out on the water, pleasure in the exercise, pleasure in handling the oars, pleasure in the sense of movement, pleasure in the sounds that are full of pictorial suggestion.[17]

However, a soldier was unable to row without the presence of a coxswain, and this is when ladies from Bedford College came to assist. Dark sets the scene:

> In the summertime a whole army of girls regularly got up early in the morning to steer the St. Dunstan's boats for an hour or two before going on to their shops and offices.
>
> Any summer morning in the years of the war there might be seen on the Regent's Park Lake two or three hundred young men in shorts and sweaters full of eager life, looking forward to the future with the courage and the certainty that should characterise youth – all of them blind, and all of them a few months before, despondent, hopeless, broken.[18]

Pearson was an enthusiastic dancer, and amongst the men he identified many who excelled at this activity. The outcome was that two dances were held every week, sometimes in a marquee on the lawn, with competitions in which famous dancers of the day were invited to act as judges and present the prizes. Pearson:

> Dancing became one of the most popular diversions with the blinded soldiers. [They] … took up dancing with astonishing zest. How well they danced was remarkable. It was a genuine source of pleasure to them, a spontaneous outlet for that spirit of enjoyment which they found, after all, had not been lost. For partners the men had the willing help of the VADs – 'Sisters' as the soldiers always called them, and the lady coxswains.[19]

According to Fraser, 'Soon, dance fever gripped St Dunstan's, and even some of the old soldiers were caught taking secret lessons.'[20]

Football was tried, with a bell placed inside the ball so that the blind men could locate its whereabouts, 'but the experiment never went further than causing some amusement'. Similarly, 'Pushball', in which a team of men attempted to push a 10-foot tall rubber ball the length of a field, and in between their opponents' (padded) goal posts, was not a great success.[21] Nevertheless, goal shooting was popular.

So much for the body; what about the mind? The Chief was a great communicator, so nothing was more natural than for him to make a point of addressing the men, on a regular basis, on current topics of interest. He also invited other people from outside of St Dunstan's to come and talk to the men. In addition, a debating society was formed, at which Pearson usually took the chair.

Music was a feature of St Dunstan's life; the moving spirit behind this being Lady Pearson. Concerts were held, in which professional instrumentalists and singers of the highest rank gave their services. However, the men were anxious to produce their own music. Fraser stated that Lady Pearson

> ... encouraged St Dunstaners to learn, to play, to perform ... So we had, at various times, a brass band, a string band, a jazz band, and a full orchestra. We had performers on every known instrument, from the double bass to the penny whistle.[22]

Finally, 'a very able concert party of blind musicians' was formed, whose, 'ceaseless round of engagements' raised considerable sums for the upkeep of St Dunstan's.[23]

The *St. Dunstan's Review*, a record of the life of Dunstan's, was written in the main by the men themselves. Produced monthly, it became a connecting link between St Dunstaners and those concerned with their welfare in all parts of the world.[24] The *Review* contained articles on such topics as rowing on the lake, Visitors' Day, horseback riding, poetry, trout fishing and golf. It also contained a parody of Rudyard Kipling's poem 'If'. This particular version, written by one of the blinded officers, appeared in the *St Dunstan's Review* of March 1917. It began:

> If you should lose your sight while all about you
> Are keeping theirs, as soldiers often do;
> If you're alive when Huns have tried to rout you,
> And do not grumble when all's lost to view...

And it ended:

> If you can keep some hens, and never scare them,
> Of eggs you'll find you need not fear a dearth;
> If you can mend old boots, and people wear them,
> You'll feel you've made your mark upon this earth.
> If you get lost, make casts like any huntsman's;
> If you feel hopeless in the dark, don't mind,

For when you've been a few months at St. Dunstan's,
You'll be a man, old chap, although you're blind.

Favourite games were chess, draughts, dominoes and cards. The black draughts were smaller than the white, in order that the men might distinguish between them, and on reaching the other side of the board, instead of placing one draught on top of another as a sighted person would, a 'double draught' was used. The dominoes had raised, instead of recessed bumps. The cards were each marked in the corner with an appropriate number of raised Braille dots. Bridge was played with a sighted player who read out the name of each card as it was played.[25] On Monday evenings there was a domino competition with prizes for the winners.

Pearson paints a delightful picture of Sundays, which, after church service, were set aside for rest and relaxation. This was the day for taking a walk, if the weather permitted. It was also

> ... a great day for polishing off letters, and a man often remained firmly tapping at a typewriter till he had finished five or six long epistles, while others would make their way to the Outer Lounge and sit in comfortable armchairs round the big fire, or in the summer under the mulberry tree on the lawn.[26]

On the afternoon of 19 April 1915, St Dunstan's received a visit from HRH Queen Alexandra (Queen consort of the late King Edward VII), Princess Victoria, the Princess Royal and Princess Maud. Queen Alexandra talked to the men, paid a visit to the workrooms, and was entertained at a concert at which all the performers were blind. She expressed her amazement at their cheerfulness and good spirits, and presented each of them with a large bunch of primroses tied with red, white and blue ribbon.

15

A Successful St Dunstan's: Aftercare

St Dunstan's' first Annual Report for the year ending 26 March 1916 announced that The Queen Mother HM Queen Alexandra had 'graciously signified her desire to become Patroness' of the organisation.[1] From that point, she would make frequent visits to St Dunstan's, often informally. The number of St Dunstaners had now risen to 150. Other notable visitors who came to boost the spirits of the blinded men in that year were the explorer Sir Ernest Shackleton and HM Queen Amelie of Portugal – who made a tour of the workshops and talked freely with the men, not realising that, when the latter were at work, such a practice was discouraged by the powers that be! On 12 July 1916, Pearson was created baronet and became Sir Arthur Pearson Bart. Also in 1916, he relinquished his interest in the *Daily Express* newspaper.

In March 1917, HM King George V visited, and took a particular interest in the poultry farm. He was followed, in May, by HRH The Prince of Wales and by HRH Princess Mary, and in the following year by HM Queen Mary, who was accompanied by Princess Mary and Prince Henry.

As the war in Europe intensified, so the numbers at St Dunstan's grew, leading to a demand for extra accommodation. It therefore became necessary, not only to obtain more property locally, but also, in Pearson's words: 'to establish centres away from London where special cases could be treated, pleasant homes where men could be sent for periods of convalescence or for holidays'.[2]

Properties obtained in 1916 included Sussex Place, three houses in Cornwall Terrace for men learning massage, Blackheath Annexe, Torquay Annexe in Devon, and more accommodation for the VADs and the relatives who came to London to visit the St Dunstaners. The following year, further properties included Holford House, Regent's Park College, a large mansion adjacent (formerly a training college for theological students) and West House at Kemp Town, Brighton, Sussex.

With regard to St Dunstan's itself – which stood in 15 acres of ground – once again, it was its owner Otto Kahn who came to the rescue. According to Pearson:

> He gave me absolute *carte blanche* to erect any buildings and effect any alterations that I thought fit to make. At the moment of writing the once beautiful gardens of St. Dunstan's are almost covered with workshops, classrooms, offices, storehouses, chapels [one Anglican and one Roman Catholic] and recreation rooms, while additions to the house extend on all sides, and the vast building which we call the Bungalow Annexe covers one of the fields.[3]

This included men's dormitories, a dispensary, a tobacco store, pensions department offices, offices of the Settlement Department (responsible for placing men in suitable positions of employment) and the Aftercare Department, and the Secretary's offices where, 'with the help of a large staff, an immense correspondence is conducted'.[4]

A single-storey wooden building, to be used as one of the men's dormitories, was donated by Lady Beatty, wife of Admiral Beatty, Commander of the 1st Battlecruiser Squadron and from 1916, Commander-in-Chief of the Grand Fleet.

Just before he lost his sight completely, Pearson had said to his wife: 'I shall soon be blind, but I will never be *a* blind man, I am going to be *the* blind man.'[5] Now, he could claim, with justification, that he had achieved his aim, for he declared St Dunstan's to be the largest concern over which he had ever presided; larger even than his newspaper and publishing empire. It should be mentioned, however, that Pearson was not alone in shouldering the responsibility for St Dunstan's, in that he had an executive council, together with medical specialists and others to advise him.

When a man left St Dunstan's, this was by no means the end of the story. Not only did the organisation continue to offer him practical help, but Pearson himself was assiduous in keeping in touch by letter, both with the St Dunstaner and his relatives, whether in Britain, or elsewhere in the world. They, for their part, were delighted to reciprocate. The man was provided with a complete set of tools, appropriate to the trade which he had been taught. If he was married, he was given a weekly allowance for the period of one year, to assist him in the payment of his rent until he became established. It was also the duty of St Dunstan's Settlement Department to find a suitable home and working premises for him, if required. Thereafter, he became the responsibility of the Aftercare Department, headed by Ian Fraser.

Captain Ian Fraser was wounded on 23 July 1916 at the Battle of the Somme, by a bullet to the head. After his injury he walked to the field dressing-station with his company commander, unable to see, but believing his blindness to be only temporary. From here, he was taken to a casino at Le Touquet, which had been converted into a hospital. He was then sent back to England and admitted to the Officers' Ward at the 2nd London General Hospital. He would never see again.[6]

In October 1916, at Pearson's invitation Fraser arrived at St Dunstan's to start his training and rehabilitation. Along with the other men, he learned typewriting and Braille, and for his specialist subject he chose carpentry. On 15 February 1917, Pearson wrote to Fraser's mother: 'I have had long talks with Ian lately, and have decided to train him up to assist me in working for the benefit of the blind.'[7] To this end, Fraser spent a month gaining experience in each of St Dunstan's different handicraft workshops.

As Pearson's assistant Fraser was given the task, in autumn 1917, of creating an aftercare department which would continue to monitor and assist, where necessary, all who had passed through St Dunstan's for the remainder of their lives. According to Sidney Dark, there were local agents throughout the United Kingdom whose task was to

... help the blind workman to obtain orders, and interest influential local people in his welfare. The raw materials are supplied at a reasonable price, and St. Dunstan's purchases large quantities of leather, willows, yarn, wood, string, twine, and so on, to supply to the boot-repairers, the basket-makers, the mat-makers, the carpenters, and the net-makers. Likewise, specialists in the various crafts paid visits to the men on a regular basis, to examine their work and to make suggestions for improvements.[8]

The following correspondence, faithfully recorded by Dark (which, he said, was a mere fraction of what Pearson received in total) demonstrates just how appreciated and respected Pearson was and the positive influence that St Dunstan's had on the men's lives. Private W. H. J. Oxenham recalled the time when he was newly blinded and in hospital:

> I then thought that I was more or less no more good for this world, but I soon began to realise my error, and as time went on and I arrived at St. Dunstan's this became more confirmed than ever, and I feel now full of confidence for the future.

Lieutenant Walter Millard declared that he was never happier than when he was

> ... at good old St. Dunstan's. Nor are those days over, for you still keep so well in touch with us who have left that we feel that we are merely away on week-end holiday and have only to walk into the place to have it at our finger-ends.

Private F. C. Fleetwood explained that his wife had gone to market that day with 'mats and netted articles' that he had made. He said, 'I hope she will sell out,' and then dryly:

> I wonder how many of us fellows have a shot at getting their own dinner. To-day I am looking after a big fire, several pots and pans, doing a bit of baking, giving to the dog his dinner, and doing a bit of matting into the bargain.

Despite the multitasking, he confessed that he was enjoying fulfilling the role of housewife! The mother of a blinded Australian soldier wrote to tell Pearson that she was grateful to him

> ... for the way my brave blind boy is able to get about so well and cheerfully, and my thanks to all those dear, kind people of St. Dunstan's, who made life so pleasant for him when the darkest of shadows had threatened to overcast his life.[9]

Pearson spoke of letters which he had received from professional men who had returned to work; from businessmen who had recommenced their 'important commercial undertakings'; from craftsmen who were earning livings comparable to sighted men in the same field of industry; from masseurs, 'who are not only securing for themselves a comfortable competency, but are doing great good to others'; from poultry farmers who had created successful smallholdings; from men who had found employment as secretaries or telephone exchange operators, and who worked 'with a skill which is scarcely believable'. Many of these letters said

> ... things about the work of St. Dunstan's which come straight from the hearts of those who have benefited by it, and go straight to the hearts of those who have been privileged to be responsible for its initiation and management.

This led Pearson to muse:

> Does anyone in the world, I wonder, receive so many delightful letters as I do? The post brings me a never-ending stream of them from all parts of the United Kingdom and of the British Empire, telling of lives filled with undreamt of happiness, and of success truly marvellous, such as has never been won by blinded men before.[10]

He revealed just how moved he was to receive such good tidings from his St Dunstaners:

> Often there comes to my mental vision a picture of the writers as I first met them, hopeless, despairing, and unable to imagine that any good thing was left for them in life. And then I see in my mind's eye these happy, resolute, competent men, who, in spite of their handicap, are showing that they can do their fair share in the work of the world. It is a picture of joyous contemplation the like of which can, I think, have been given to few to conjure up.[11]

Such heartfelt gratitude from his men, and more importantly the knowledge that they had 'made good', were to Pearson the greatest reward that he could have wished for.

16

Gladys Cooper, the Fresh Air Fund and St Dunstan's

English actress and beauty of the day Gladys Constance Cooper was one of many celebrities who helped Pearson fundraising, not only for St Dunstan's but also for his Fresh Air Fund. Born at Lewisham, Kent, on 18 December 1888, Gladys's father Charles F. W. Cooper, was a journalist and founding editor of *The Epicure* – a pioneering food and drink magazine. Her mother was Mabel (née Barnett). Gladys acknowledged that her parents 'belonged to the literary and artistic set of their day'. As for herself, she declared: 'I do not think I had any stage heredity in me, yet I suppose I must have always possessed, unconsciously, a sense of drama.'[1]

It was a friend of Gladys's, Mary Henessey – herself an aspiring actress – who encouraged Gladys to go for a 'voice trial' at London's Vaudeville Theatre in the Strand. The outcome was that, in 1905, Gladys made her stage debut, touring with British actor, playwright, theatre manager and producer Seymour Hicks in his musical *Bluebell in Fairyland*. From this she went on to pantomime, before joining theatre manager George Edwardes at London's Gaiety Theatre in 1907.

Gladys was sent for by Charles Hawtrey and offered a part in W. Somerset Maugham's play *The Noble Spaniard*. On 12 December 1908, she married Herbert J. Buckmaster at St George's, Hanover Square. The couple set up home in a small flat in London's Baker Street, where Gladys had her first child, Joan, born 5 July 1910. In May 1911, Gladys returned to the stage in her first 'straight part' in a play called *Half a Crown* at the Royalty Theatre. She said, 'Work tumbled my way just about this time.'[2]

In 1911, Gladys was engaged by actor and manager George Alexander to play Cecily Cardew in Oscar Wilde's *The Importance of Being Earnest* at the St James's Theatre. She then appeared in a variety of plays – including ones by George Bernard Shaw and John Galsworthy – at various theatres including The Royalty, Drury Lane and Wyndhams.

In 1913, Gladys appeared in her first film, Adolph Zukor's *The Eleventh Commandment* (1913). The year or so before the First World War said Gladys, was 'the best I have ever known'.[3] During the War, Gladys's husband Herbert Buckmaster served for three and a half years on the Western Front as an officer in the 12th Reserve Regiment of Cavalry. Meanwhile, Gladys continued with her acting career: 'The play that people seem to remember me best in is *My Lady's Dress*', which was produced in 1914.[4] In late 1914, Gladys travelled with Seymour Hicks and his company to France, where they gave concerts to the British, French, and Belgian troops.

Gladys had met Sir Arthur prior to the War, and it was through him that she had become associated with the Fresh Air Fund. It was to Sir Arthur, she said, that she

> … had been of assistance occasionally in some of his philanthropic schemes. On one occasion when he gave a very big ball at the Savoy for the benefit of the blind men of St Dunstan's, I was able to be of very considerable help to him, and sold heaps of tickets and got a very large number of people interested. As everyone knows, St Dunstan's was the entire work and creation of Sir Arthur Pearson. Blind himself, he had the keenest sympathy and the tenderest understanding of the sufferings and deprivations of the blind.[6]

She described the ball as 'the finest I have ever been to', and said of Pearson:

> There is no doubt that he is a wonderful man. He was completely blind, but he had a marvellous way of looking after himself. He knew, for example, exactly where his tea-cup could be safely put at the edge of a table, and he never seemed to fumble with things. We frequently talked about being blind, and I remember once saying to him, 'I can't begin to understand what it means – I can't enter into things with blind people as you can,' and him

replying, 'Ah, but then, you see, I am *with* the blind.' That was what he always said to other blind men: 'I am *with* you.'⁵

Knowing of Gladys's love of children, Sir Arthur wrote to her and asked if she would write an article for one of his newspapers in connection with the Fresh Air Fund. This, said Gladys, 'was a charity after my own heart,' and she would be delighted 'to get some poor mites a happy country outing'.⁷ The only other woman, besides herself, that Sir Arthur approached to write on behalf of the fund was Ellaline Terriss, star of musical comedies. Whereas Terriss contributed to *Pearson's Magazine*, Gladys wrote for *The Royal Magazine* (launched on 14 October 1898 by C. Arthur Pearson): 'I hope as long as I live to be associated with these two great philanthropic schemes.'

In July 1915, Gladys's son John was born but within a few weeks she had returned to the stage – cast as an 'American witch' in *The Real Thing At Last*, a film parody of Shakespeare's play *Macbeth* by A.E. Matthews. The film was launched at a Royal Command Performance in aid of British troops on 7 March 1916 at the London Coliseum.

In 1927, Gladys (who had divorced from Herbert Buckmaster) married Sir Neville Pearson, Sir Arthur's son. As far as the Fresh Air Fund was concerned, Gladys was as good as her word. She was present, for example, on 23 June 1931, when HRH The Duke of Kent (later King George VI) joined celebrations in Epping Forest, Essex, marking the 40th year of the Fund.

17

Pearson's
Winning Formula

One of the many evocative images of St Dunstan's is that of the blind boot-repairers singing the 'Cobblers' Song' at the top of their voices as they worked. But how could it possibly be that men who had survived the ordeal of the battlefield, and who, on top of everything else, now had to contend with being blind, were so happy? These men had gone to war as members of the British Empire; as potential conquering heroes. Yet they had returned battered, bloodied and bruised, with the added disappointment of having failed in their objective of achieving a speedy victory. Not only that, but having been blinded in battle, their last, most vivid, and most enduring memories would have been horrific ones. And how did it come about that, in Fraser's words: 'Between 90 and 95 per cent of those who passed through St Dunstan's could – and did – earn a living, or at any rate, add substantially to their pensions after they had left.' And this, after only a few months of training – a truly astonishing achievement.[1]

Psychological Support

During the First World War, as many as five per cent of soldiers were removed from the battlefield because they were suffering from shell-shock

– otherwise known as 'war neurosis'. This condition (which today would be called 'post-traumatic stress disorder') was characterised by depression, excessive irritability, guilt (at having survived, when so may others had not), recurrent nightmares, flashbacks to traumatic scenes and over–reaction to sudden noises.

In the first year of the War, many of the victims of shell-shock were regarded as insane. As the War progressed, it was recognised by the army medical officers and specialist nurses that what such patients required was rest, quiet and relaxation. It was not until 1917 that intensive six-week courses were arranged to teach medical officers how to recognize and how to treat shell-shock casualties in the forward battle areas. Those at St Dunstan's who were suffering from shell-shock would undoubtedly have received the same care and treatment.

It is significant that Pearson makes no mention of the word 'psychologist' in his book *Victory over Blindness* – a record of life and work at St Dunstan's. Even its penultimate chapter – entitled 'The Psychology of the Blinded Soldier' – was written, not by a psychologist, but by author and journalist Richard King Huskinson q.v., who was also one of St Dunstan's volunteer helpers.

A Convivial Atmosphere

In the armed services, the men had been subjected to strict discipline with an overwhelming array of rules and regulations. St Dunstan's also had its rules, and if a man broke them he was disciplined. If the breach was sufficiently serious, he was asked to leave the organisation. However, in the main the atmosphere was overwhelmingly one of warmth and conviviality.

One of the pleasures that the men enjoyed, both in the services and at St Dunstan's was a cigarette or a pipe of tobacco, and as Pearson said:

> Visitors to the hostel were generally surprised to find that the habit of smoking was almost universal among the men. Certainly one of the pleasures of smoking is lost to one who cannot see the smoke, yet it remains not only a pleasure but a solace to the blinded man. At St Dunstan's the men smoked at work as well as at other times. Pipes were not commonly used; it was the cigarette that was popular.[2]

Spiritual Support

The spiritual needs of the men were catered for by an Anglican or a Roman Catholic clergyman who conducted the church services on Sundays. In addition, chaplains were always on hand to talk to the men.

Blind Teachers

Both Pearson and the men knew how important it was, psychologically, for the blind where possible, to be taught by blind teachers:

> When a blinded man with that horrible feeling of helplessness which first overcomes him, particularly if he tries to do something, finds that the man who is teaching him is blind himself, he thinks at once: 'I am not being asked to do something which is impossible, by someone who does not understand. I am being shown the right way – this man who is blind knows what he is doing and I too can do it.[3]

To this end, if a trainee at St Dunstan's was found to have a particular aptitude for teaching, and to possess sufficient skill in his craft, then he was swiftly recruited into the ranks of the teaching staff.

The Danger of Mollycoddling

Pearson encouraged family members to visit the men and facilitated their doing so by paying their railway train or omnibus fares, and inviting them to stay for a few days, or even for a week, at the organisation's expense. When the visitors arrived, the 'Chief' was quick to explain his ideas to them:

> I had sometimes to insist that a newly blinded man's worst enemy was apt to be his own loving wife, or mother, or sister. For the tender desire to wait on a blinded man, to do everything for him, to remove all difficulties from his path, has the effect of preventing him from making the wonderful discovery of all he can do for himself.

To the public I say: do not pity these blinded men, give them all the sympathy in the world, give them all the help you possibly can, encourage them in their growing spirit of independence; when you walk with them guide them as little as possible, when you talk to them do not talk to them as men cut off from all the beauty of the world and of the passing interests of the day. If they have set themselves to forget what they have suffered and what they are suffering, is it for you to remind them?[4]

In other words, family and friends, however well meaning, could easily undo all the good work done by St Dunstan's, and in doing so prevent a man's recovery rather than facilitating it. On the positive side, relatives were invited to participate in parts of the relevant training courses themselves. This was because there were aspects of certain occupations which required that sighted assistance be given to the blind man.

The Women

Women were another vital factor, and Pearson himself was fulsome in his praise of the multitude of females – including the dedicated nursing staff – who played such a pivotal role in the rehabilitation process. In fact, even before the men had arrived at St Dunstan's he noted: 'The soldier who had lost his sight was given most tender care by the Sisters, Superintendents and Nurses [in the hospitals in which they found themselves]'.[5]

And later, at St Dunstan's:

One thinks of the women workers especially – of how they contributed to the happiness of the men, of how they gladdened their hearts, taking the trouble to understand them, and to bring just the right kind of cheer and sympathy to bear on their problems.

Pearson acknowledged that most of the work of St Dunstan's was 'gladly undertaken' by women. The VADs, for example

... supervised the men's arrivals, departures, and holidays. They organised cars and trains to take them to the theatre; on excursions – for they received many invitations in the outside world – and on week-end outings. They occupied themselves in reading letters, or opening parcels which the men received in the post. Writing letters for them when the need arose; reading aloud to them, and, in short, helping in every way to entertain them in their hours of leisure.

Women also attended to the laundry, darned socks, undertook sewing repairs, made the beds, did the housework and waited on the men at table. As the St Dunstan's organisation grew in size, there were eventually some 600 women who 'devoted all or a great part of their time to this labour of love', the majority being volunteers.

As for Matron, just as the men viewed Pearson as a father figure, so equally they regarded her as a mother. (In fact, to many who were 'mere lads,' said Pearson, she was 'the Supreme Mother'.) The same applied to the sisters, and trained nurses who presided over the dispensaries. They did so, 'with a mother's care and more than a mother's skill'.[6]

The female secretary, who dealt with administration also earned the men's devotion. In fact, in all the offices of St Dunstan's there were 'women doing work on which ... the happiness of the men depended.'

Pearson – the 'Chief'

The original motto of St Dunstan's was somewhat uninspiring: 'What the eye does not see the heart does not grieve about'. However, a new motto was adopted: 'Victory Over Blindness'. This was also the title Pearson gave to one of his books, and it epitomised his indomitable spirit. (Another of Pearson's books was entitled *Conquest Over Blindness*). For example, Sidney Dark happened to overhear a conversation in which Matron told Pearson that one of the men was despondent. 'Despondent, what on earth has he got to be despondent about?' came the reply. The word 'despondency' was, apparently, not a part of the Chief's vocabulary!

Pearson was also aware of the importance of preserving the dignity of the men, and when a blind officer asked him if 'some device could be invented to enable blind men to play billiards', he regarded this as a step too far:

For Heaven's sake, don't let us make ourselves ridiculous. Its absurd to try and play a game like billiards, which absolutely depends on keen sight. There are so many things that we can do, without making asses of ourselves.[7]

'Affliction', or 'Handicap'?

Pearson was shocked when a deputation of teachers and pupils arrived from an institution for the blind in the north of England, and its chairman referred to his blind pupils as 'the little afflicted ones'. Pearson gave this withering repost: 'If you tell a man often enough that he is afflicted he will become afflicted and will adopt the mental and physical attitude befitting that soul-destroying word.'[8]

Instead, he suggested the alternative word, 'handicap', for this was something which could be overcome, even if a handicapped person cannot perform tasks as quickly as normal.[9] Today, the word 'disability' might be seen to be more appropriate.

Pearson the Indomitable

Pearson led by example, he lived his life with characteristic gusto and refused to seek help for himself if he could possibly avoid it: 'I set myself to live as active and as independent a life as possible,' he said. He was equally determined that his men should do the same, in order that they might 'escape from that passive half-life which seemed so commonly accepted as inevitable'.[10]

According to Fraser, Pearson demonstrated his independence of spirit in typical fashion when it came to taking his meals:

> He refused all help, and claimed he could deal with anything that was put on his plate, from a lamb chop to a chicken wing. He only got away with it because jolly good care was taken to see that no bone was ever put on his plate. In fairness, I must say that this was not done with his connivance.[11]

This had unforeseen consequence, for, as Fraser describes, in attempting to follow Pearson's example one of the men became 'over-inspired', with the result that at the meal table he 'got into an awful mess trying to cut up his tie!'

Pearson was meticulous by nature, both in appearance and in his work, and he expected his men to be the same: 'People seem apt to think that if a man is blind he must necessarily be untidy. He very often is. But as St Dunstaners know, I attach the greatest importance to tidiness and smartness.'[12] There were limits, however, to what even Pearson could achieve unaided, and he freely acknowledged the help given to him by Irene Mace, his personal assistant and guide (who subsequently became Commandant of the VADs.)[13]

Inspired by Pearson's example, the men almost invariably found that they developed a new surge of interest and energy, which was accompanied by an improvement in their general health. Occasionally however, there were bad days – days of immense frustration – and it may take the encouraging words of Pearson, a VAD or Matron to dispel feelings of anger or helplessness.

Pearson's Impatience

Although Fraser describes Pearson as being 'generous and warm-hearted', there was also another side to him:

> He was quick-tempered as well as quick-witted, and if you did not see his point as quickly as he thought you should, he was liable to flare up and blow you out of the room. But the mood quickly passed, and he was never too big to apologise.[14]

Pearson, the Champion of his Men

For disabled service personnel, the awarding of pensions was in accordance with an antiquated system dating back to the year 1754 in which the Chelsea Commissioners, acting in conjunction with the Army Council, acted as adjudicators.

Up until February 1915, the maximum compensation paid to a totally blinded soldier, as a result of war service, was half a crown (two shillings and sixpence) per day, or seventeen shillings and sixpence per week.[15] By March 1915, the amount had been increased to 25 shillings per week for a private soldier, rising to up to 40 shillings per week for a warrant officer class one. In December 1916, the various pension departments were brought under the single umbrella of the Ministry of Pensions. Nonetheless, said Fraser, this system proved 'hopelessly impracticable, creating suspicion among disabled soldiers and causing lengthy delays'.[16]

The battle was now joined by Pearson who fought successfully for his blind men to receive an 'attendant allowance' in addition to their basic pension. However, the government created further problems by insisting that a blinded man must prove that his disability was directly attributable to war service. This was often impossible to do because many of the men had pre-existing eye conditions before they had even enlisted in the armed services.

A compromise was reached when pension eligibility was extended to men discharged from the Army on account of their having a pre-existing disease that had been aggravated by war service. However, because of the narrow interpretation of the word 'aggravation' by the Ministry, many legitimate claims were refused. Finally, as a result of pressure put upon it, the Ministry set up an appeals board, and later a pensions appeal tribunal. Whereupon, St Dunstan's responded by establishing its own dedicated pensions office in which it employed its own pensions officer to represent its men.[17] W. G. Askew, who was appointed Pensions Officer in 1919, was responsible for winning 85% of cases which went to the Appeals Tribunal.

In his continuing battles with the Ministry, Pearson had a staunch ally in Sir Arnold Lawson, who spoke on behalf of the men at the Pensions Appeal Tribunals, pointing out that those with defective eyesight ought never to have been admitted into the armed services in the first place. It was therefore, 'adding insult to injury for the Tribunal to disclaim responsibility for such persons'.

The fact that Pearson was prepared to go to such lengths for his men was yet another sign that in the Chief they had a resolute leader, and a steadfast and true friend in whom they could have every confidence.

There were other factors, apart from those quoted above, which made St Dunstan's the success that it undoubtedly was. Pearson had already alluded to the possibly danger of mollycoddling by the relatives and friends. There was more to it than that, however. A newly blinded man, sent straight home from hospital, rather than to St Dunstan's, finds himself in

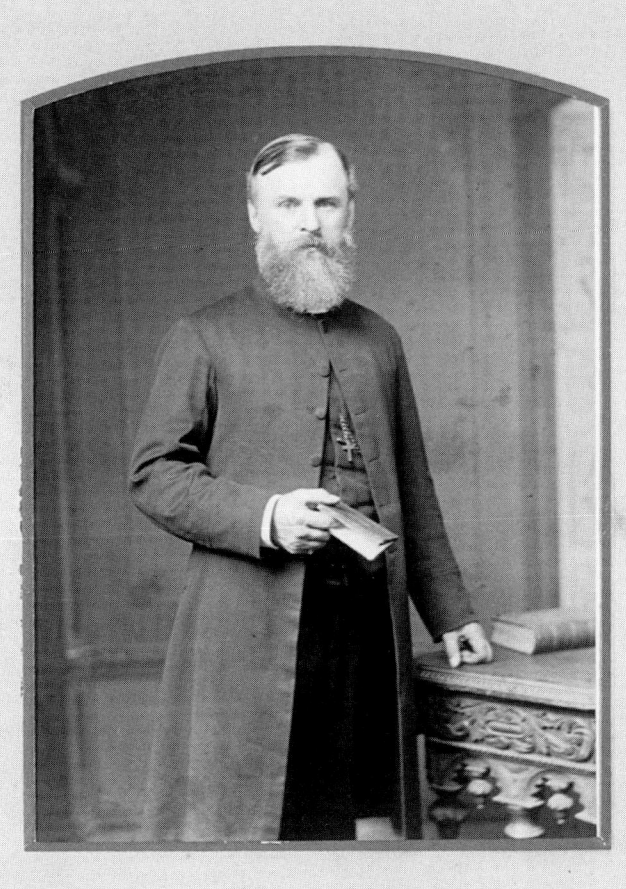

The Reverend A. Cyril Pearson, Rector of Springfield. Photo: Essex Record Office.

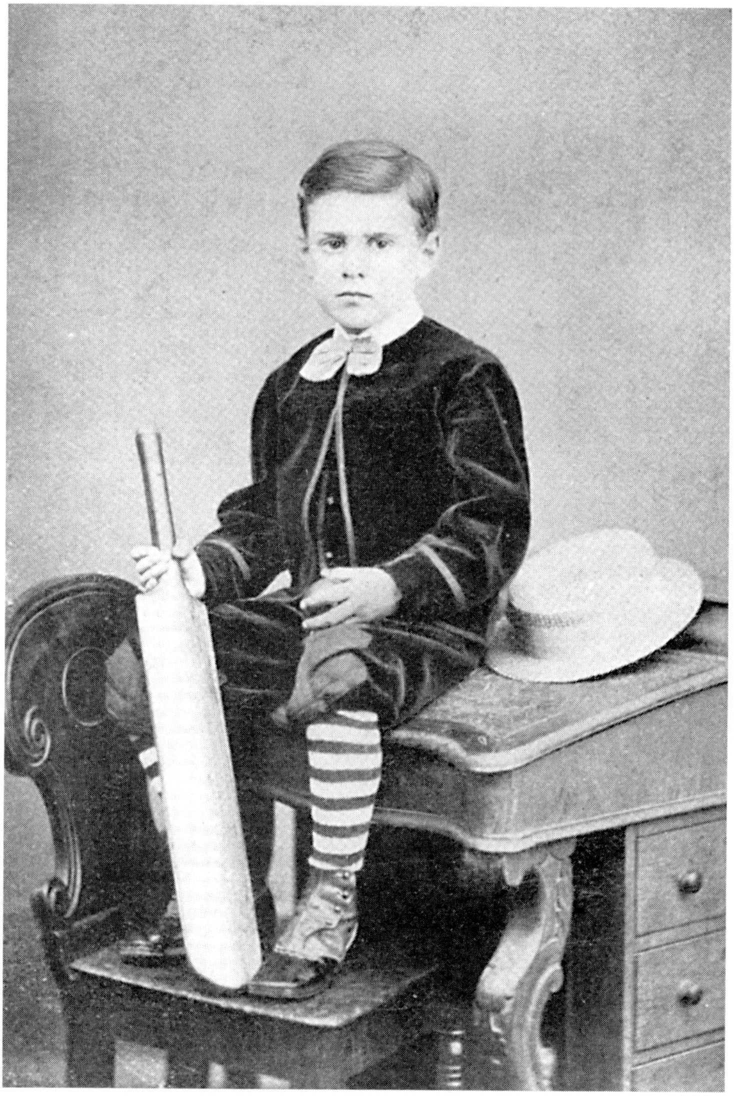

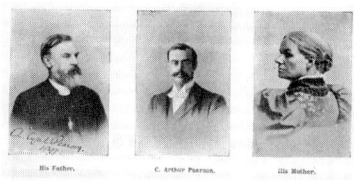

C. Arthur Pearson, 1875, aged 9. Photo: (copyright) F. Spalding.

Pearson and his parents.

Pearson's Weekly

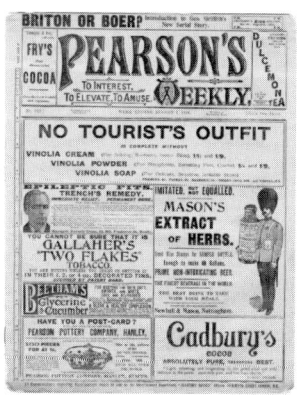

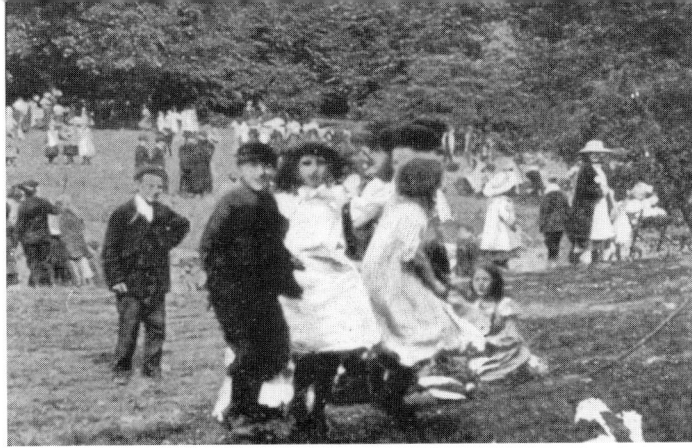

Fresh Air Fund:
Children in
Epping Forest.
Photo: Pearson's
Holiday Fund.

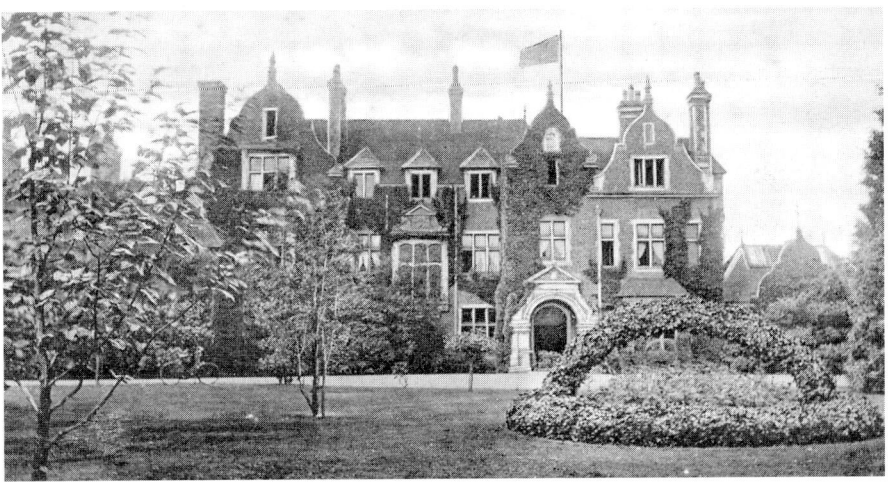

Frensham Place. Photo: Rural Life Centre, Tilford, Surrey.

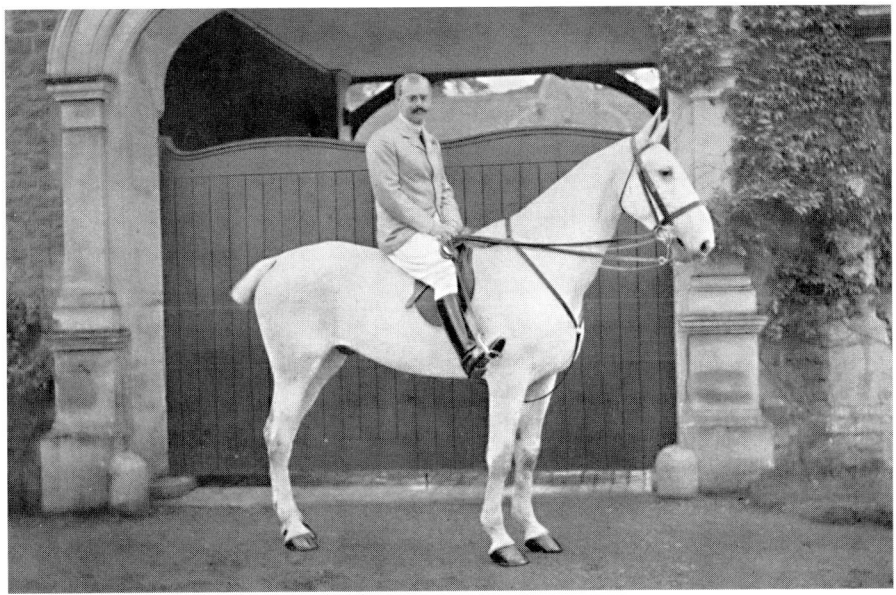

Outside the stables at Frensham Place, 1906. Photo: Hale's Studios, Farnham.

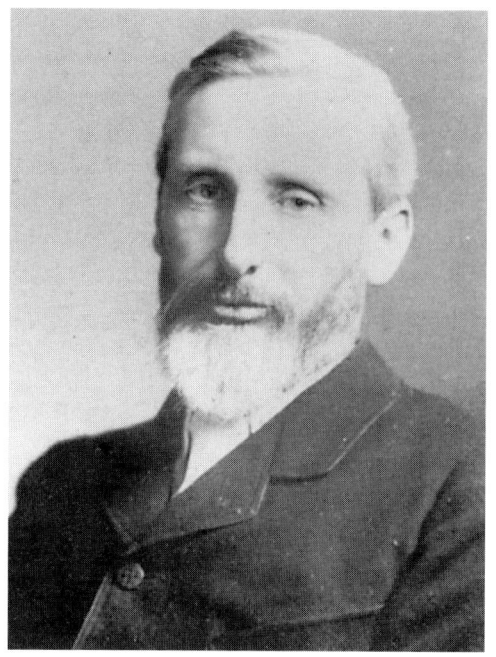

Grant Allen.

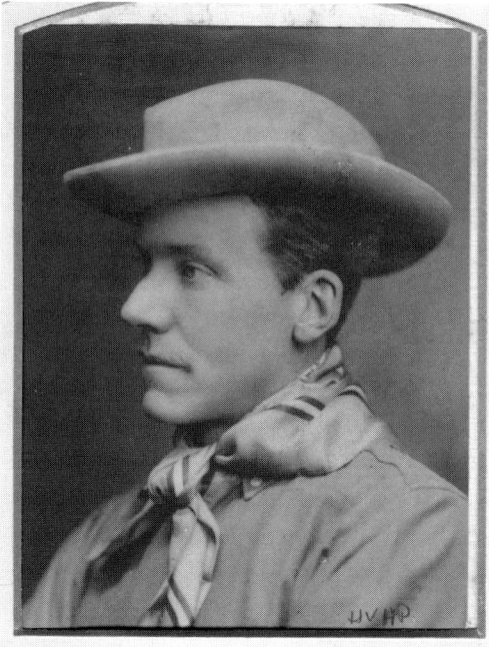

Hesketh V. H. Prichard. Photo: Charlie Jacoby.

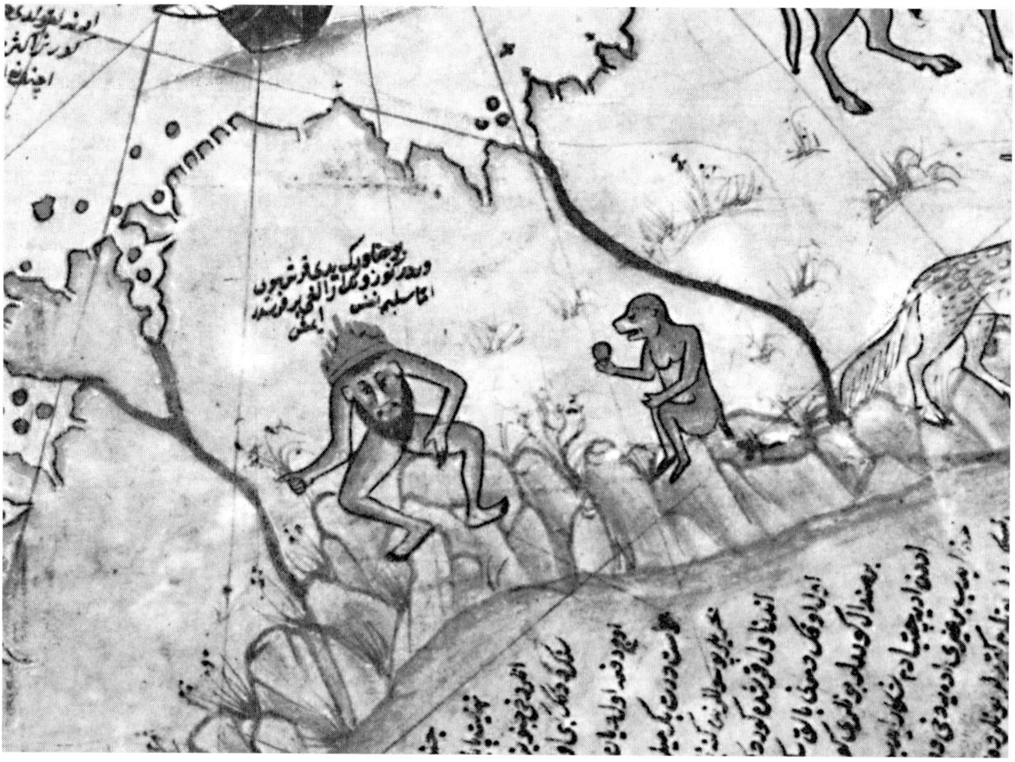

The 'dog-headed creature' from the 16th Century Piri Reis Map. Photo: Cambridge University Library.

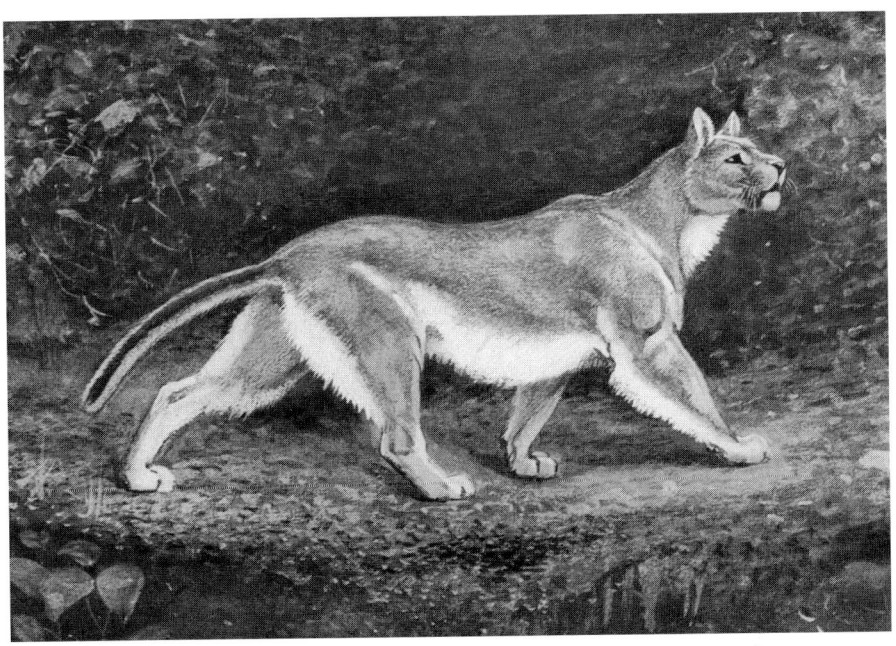

Felis concolor pearsoni – 'Pearson's Puma' by John Guille Millais.

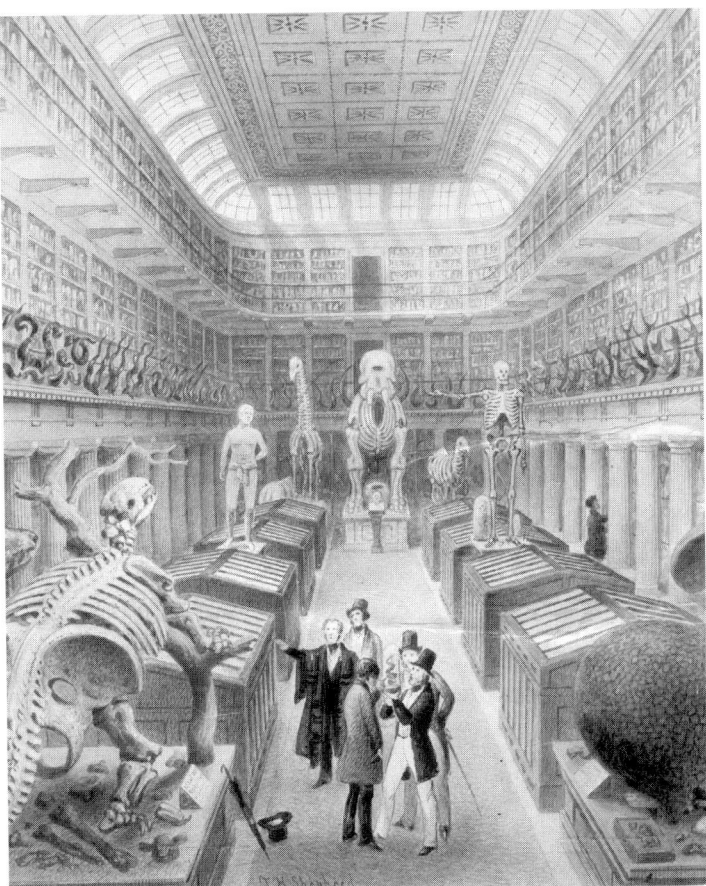

Skeleton of the Giant Sloth (left foreground) on display at the Hunterian Museum, London, circa 1860, watercolour by T. H. Shepherd. Photo: Royal College of Surgeons of England.

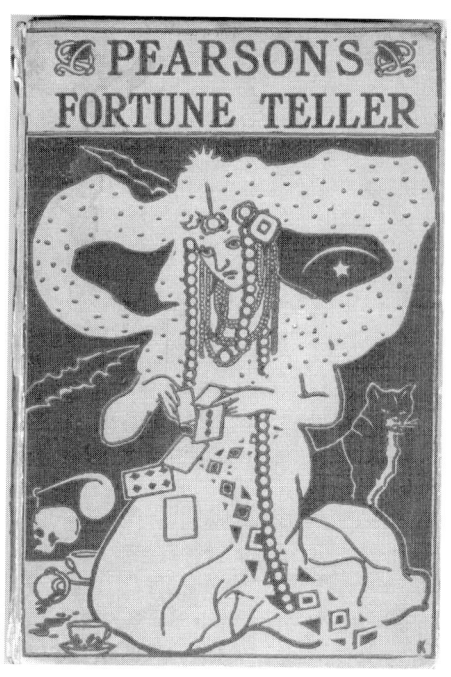

Pearson's Fortune Teller.

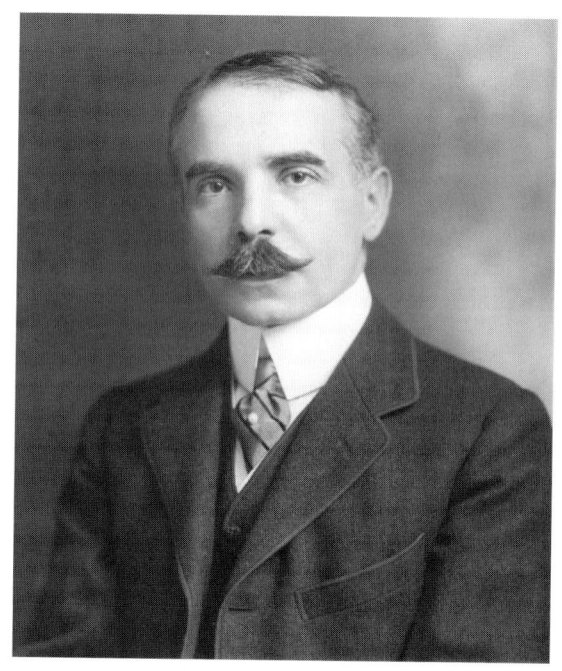

Otto Kahn.

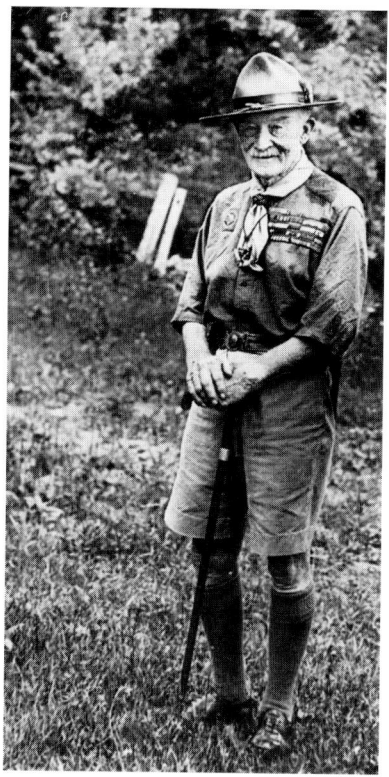

Lord Baden-Powell. Photo: The Scout Association.

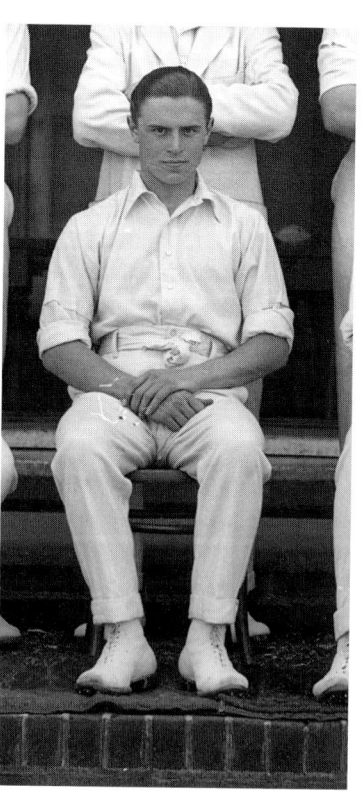

Neville Arthur Pearson, Eton XI 1915–16. Photo: M. T. Phillips, Curator, Eton College Photographic Archive.

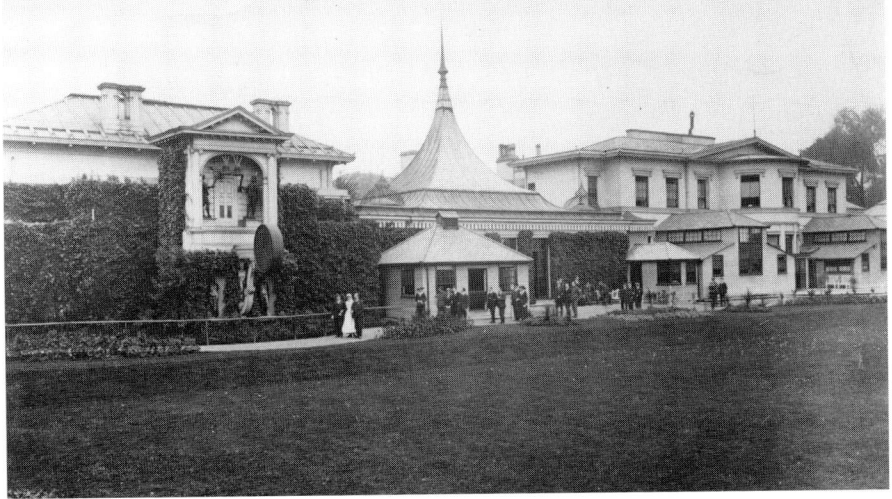

St Dunstan's Lodge, Training Centre, 1915–20. Photo: St Dunstan's.

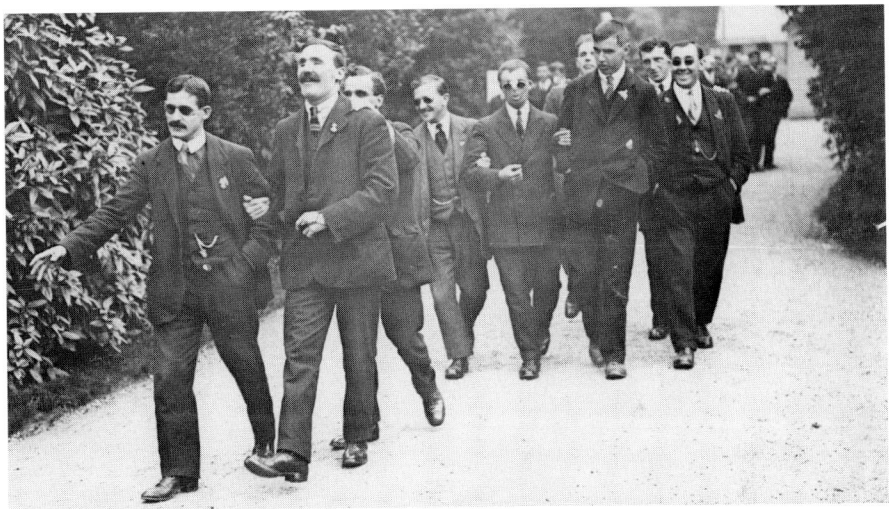

Group of early St Dunstaners. Copyright Ernest E. Smerdon. Photo: St Dunstan's.

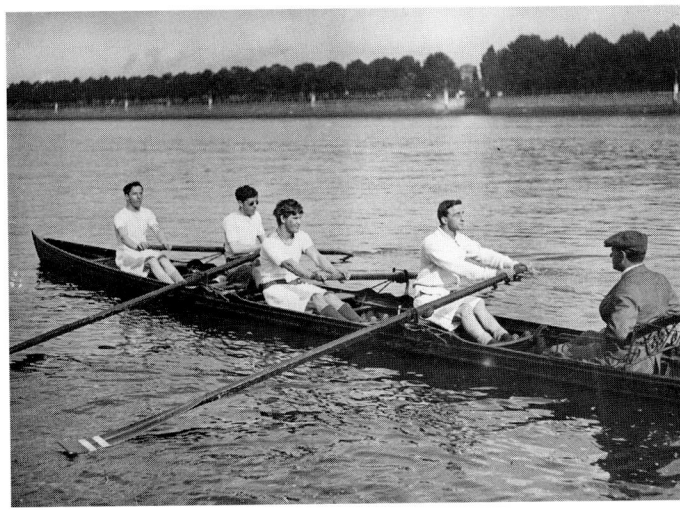

St Dunstaners Rowing
Fours on the River
Thames, 1920.
Photo: St Dunstan's.

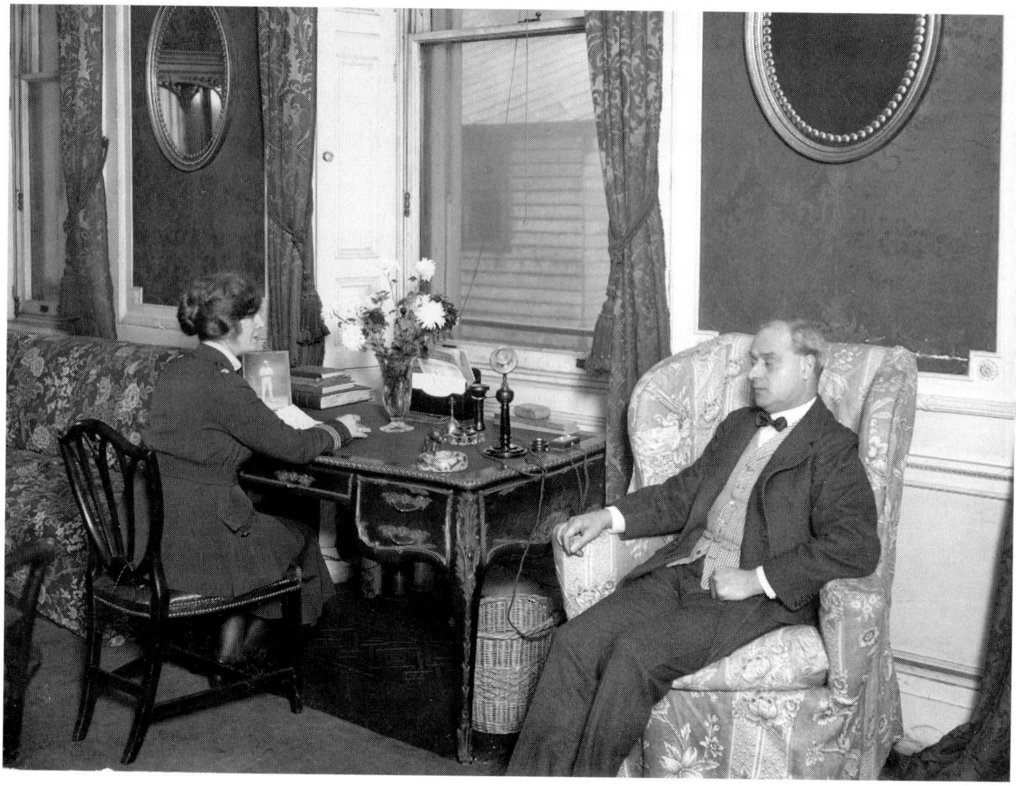

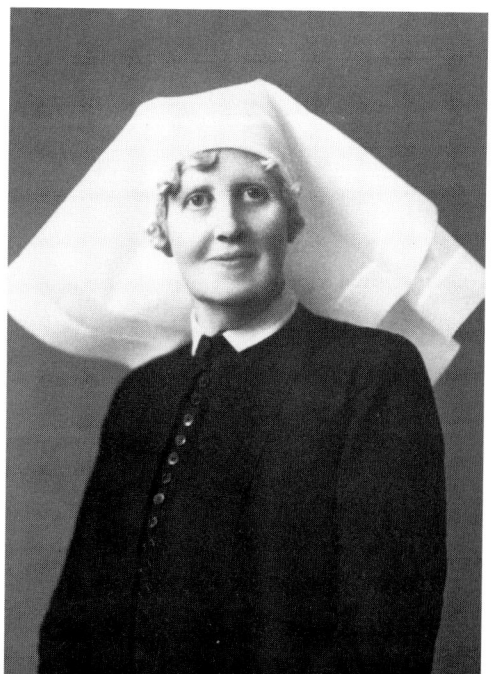

Arthur Pearson in his office in Regent's Park.
Photo: St Dunstan's.

Matron Boyd-Rochfort OBE.
Photo: St Dunstan's.

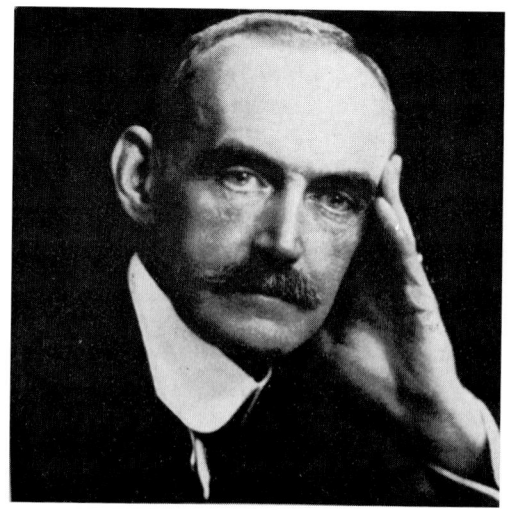

Sir Arnold Lawson. Photo: Royal College of
Ophthalmologists.

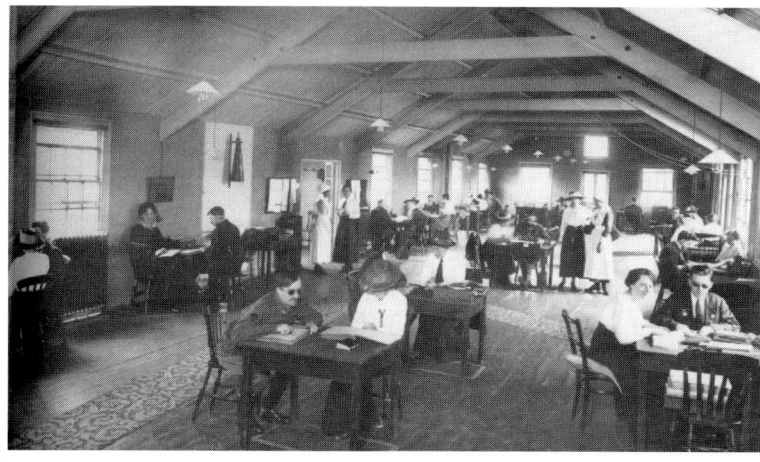

Learning Braille. Photo:
St Dunstan's.

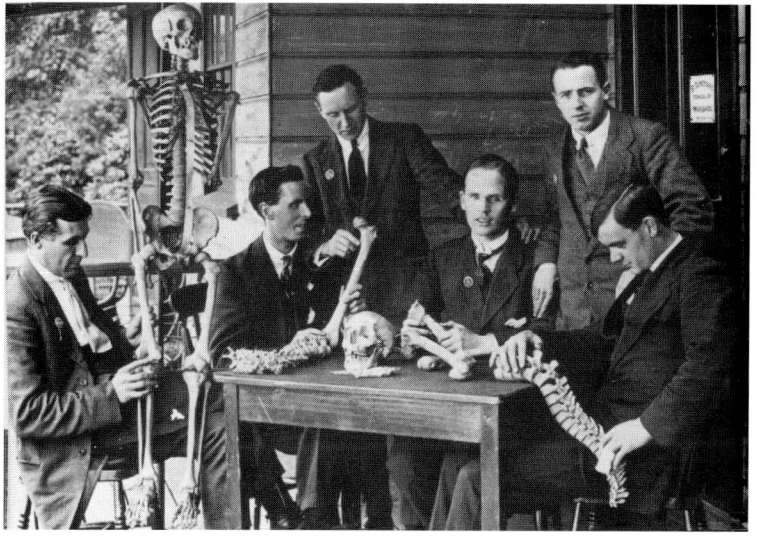

First World War masseurs in
training at St Dunstan's.
Photo: St Dunstan's.

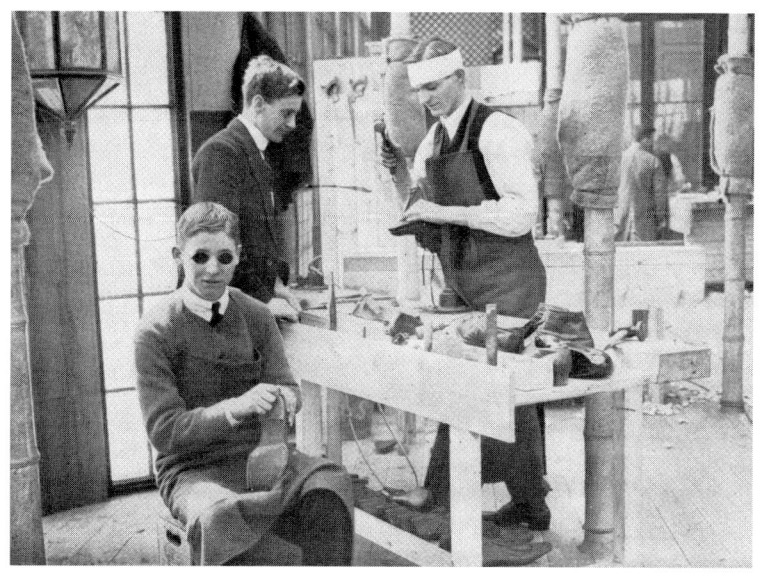

Boot repairing. Photo:
St Dunstan's.

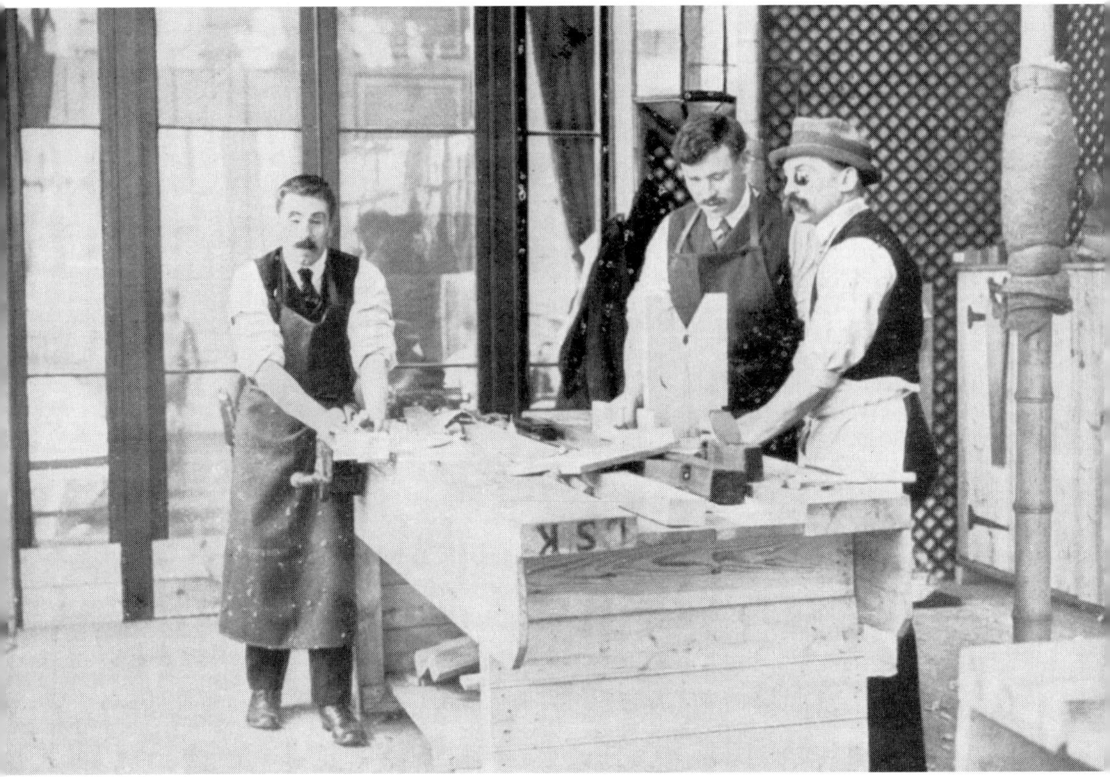

Training in joinery. Photo: St Dunstan's.

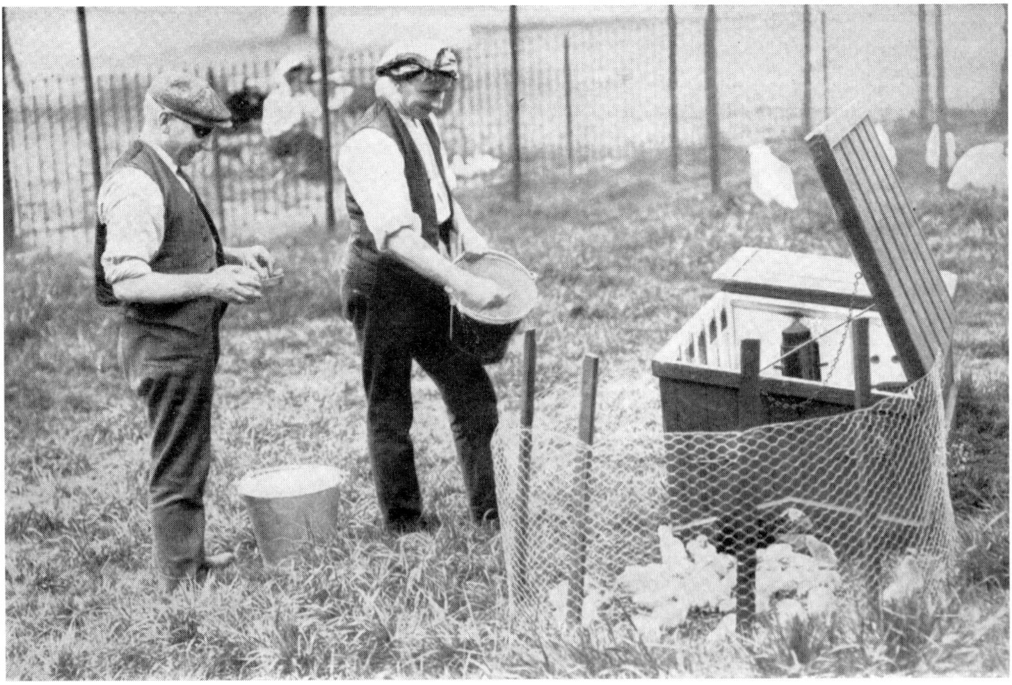

Poultry farming. Photo: (copyright) Sport and General.

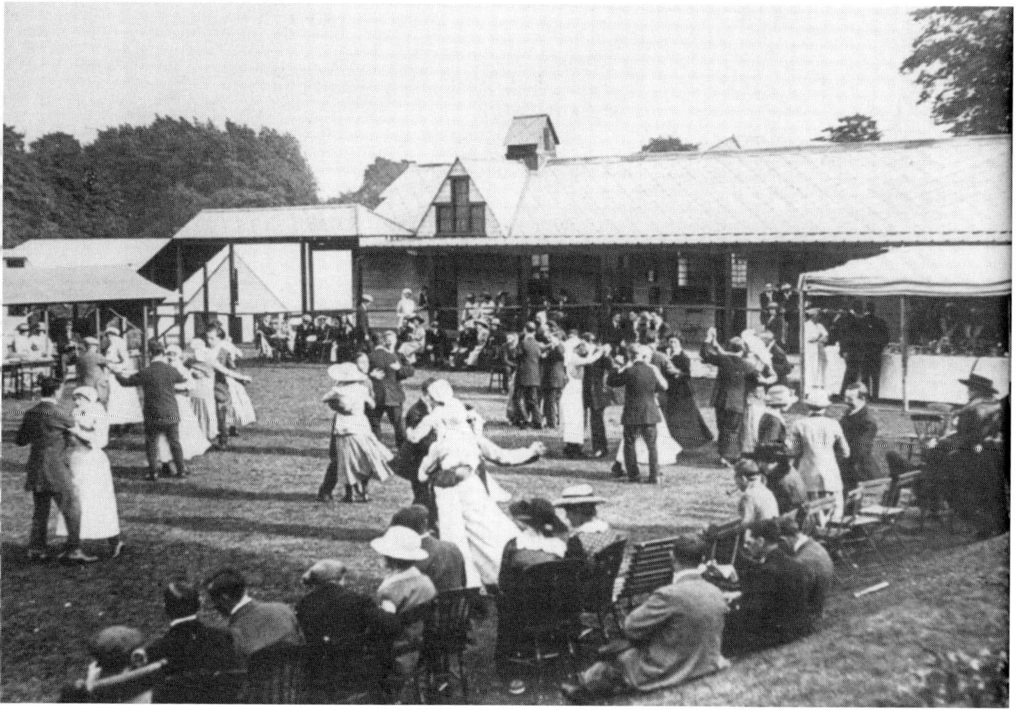

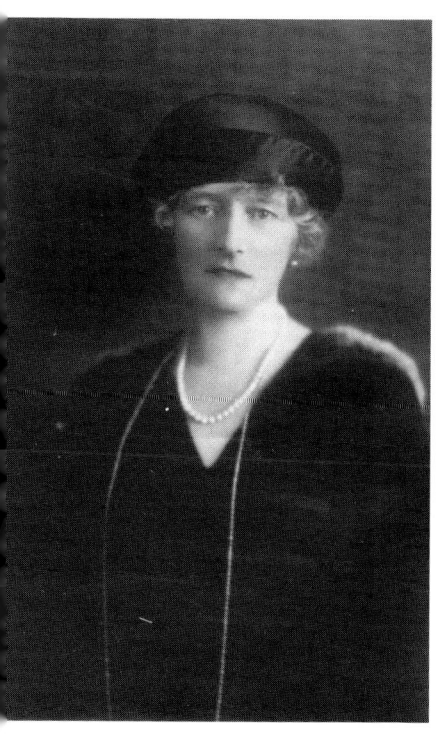

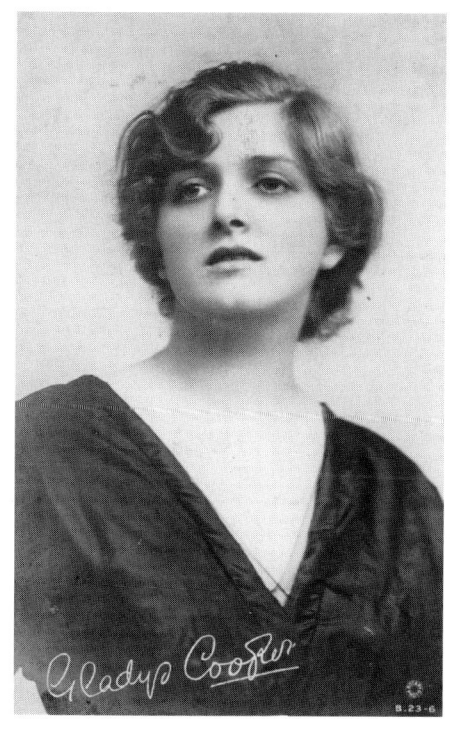

St Dunstan's, Regent's Park: dance with men, VADs and nurses. Photo: St Dunstan's.

Lady Pearson. Photo: St Dunstan's.

Gladys Cooper. Photo: Sally Hardy.

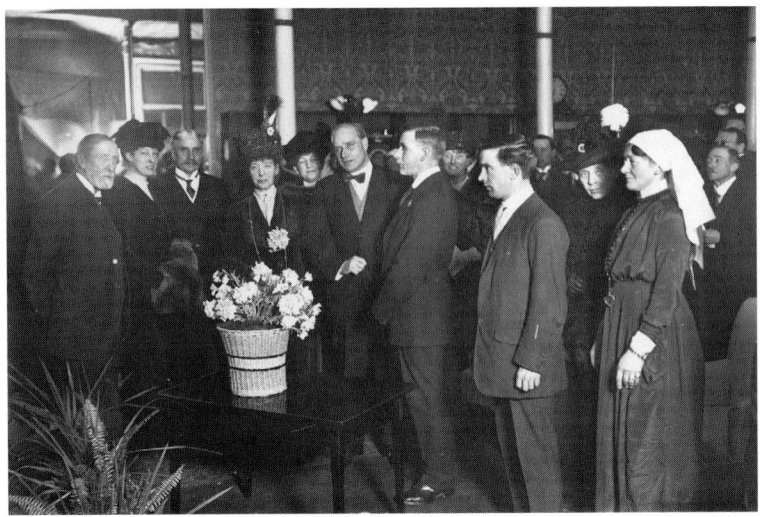

Queen Alexandra
(to left of Sir Arthur
Pearson) at St
Dunstan's Lodge,
December 1918.
Photo: St Dunstan's.

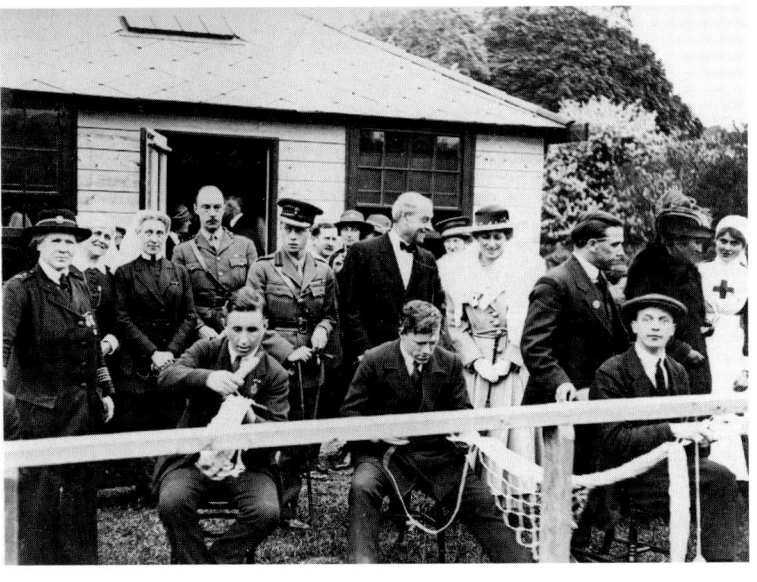

HRH The Prince
of Wales and HRH
Princess Mary at St
Dunstan's 1917. Photo:
St Dunstan's.

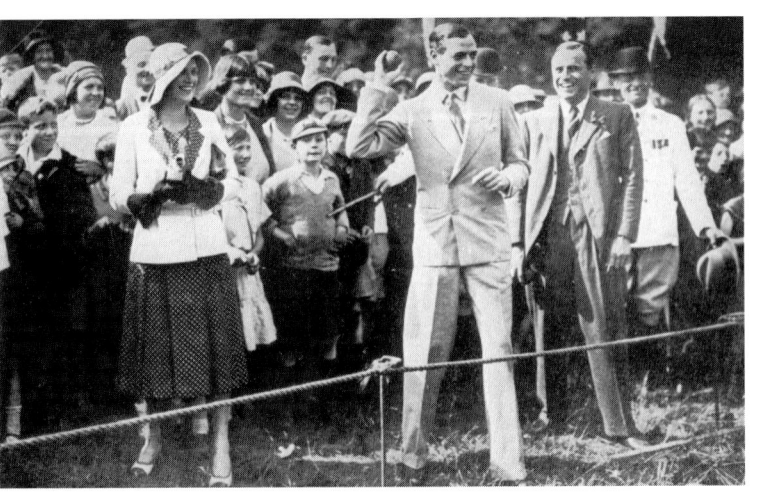

Gladys Cooper with
HRH The Duke of
Kent, opening the
Fresh Air Fund, 1931.
Photo: Sally Hardy.

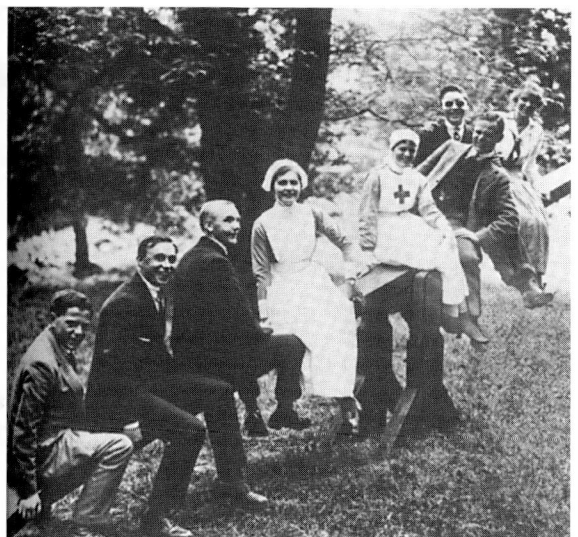

St Dunstaners with VADs.

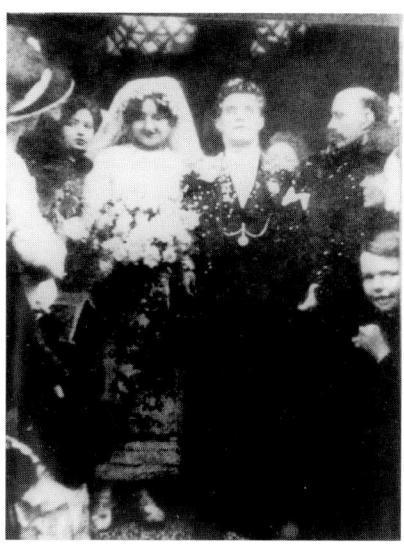

Wedding of Thomas Waldin and Esther Benwell, 26 October 1916. Photo: Jean Norman.

Thomas Waldin at work in St John's Wood, 1920. Photo: Jean Norman.

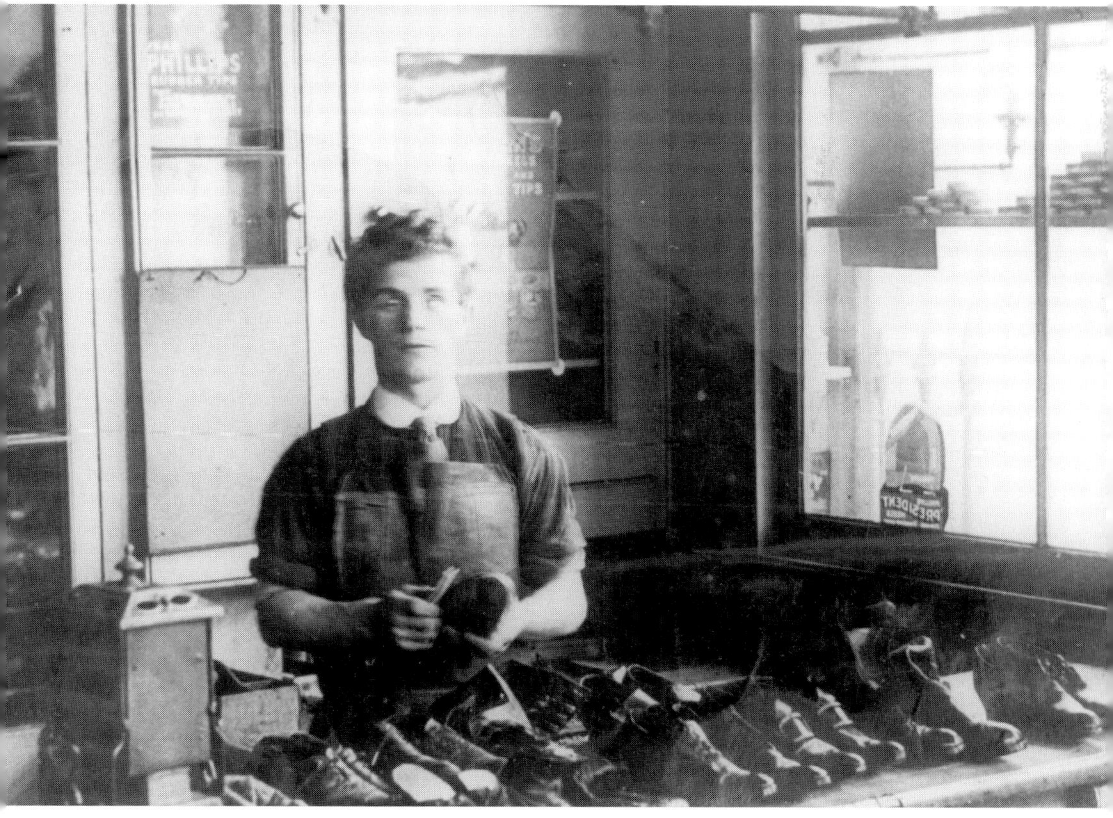

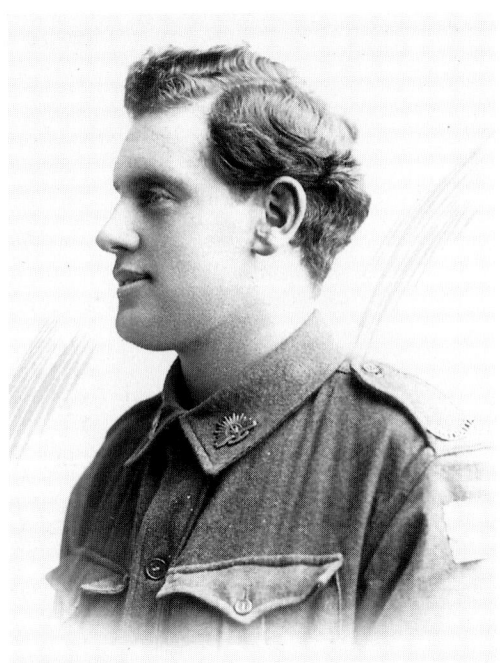

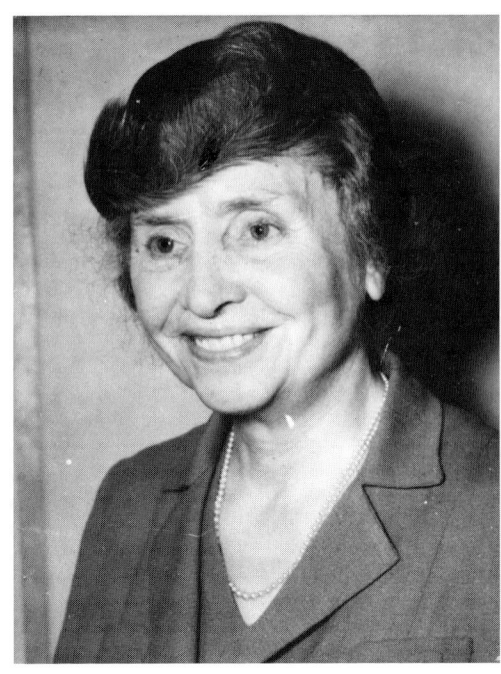

Elmer Glew. Photo: Courtesy of Vision Australia Heritage Collection.

Helen Adams Keller. Photo: Courtesy of Vision Australia Heritage Collection.

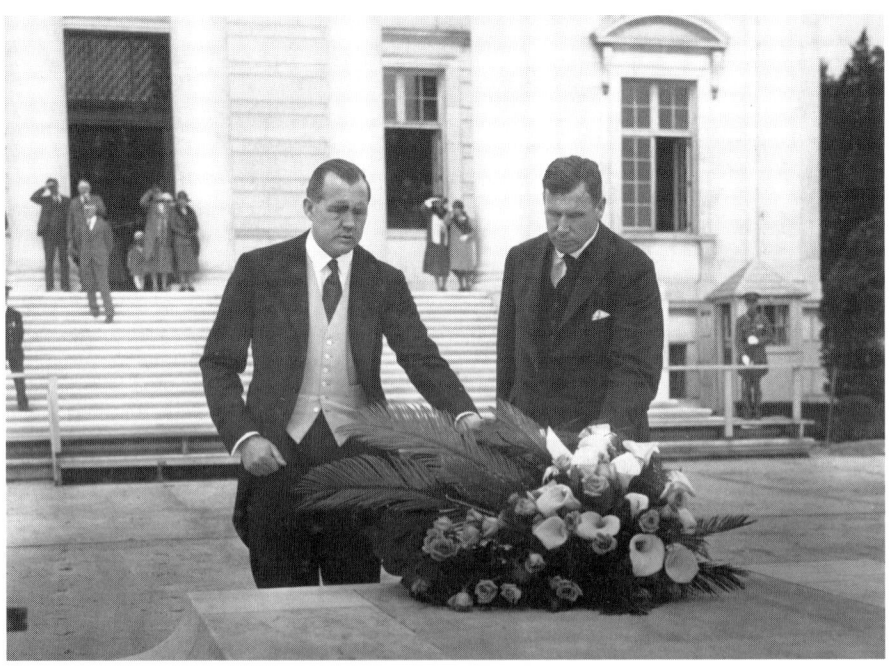

Captain Ian Fraser, CBE, Chairman of St Dunstan's, London, and Clutha MacKenzie, Director of the Jubilee Institute for the Blind of New Zealand, visiting the Tomb of the Unknown Soldier at Arlington National Cemetery, Washington DC, 1931. Photo: Royal New Zealand Foundation of the Blind.

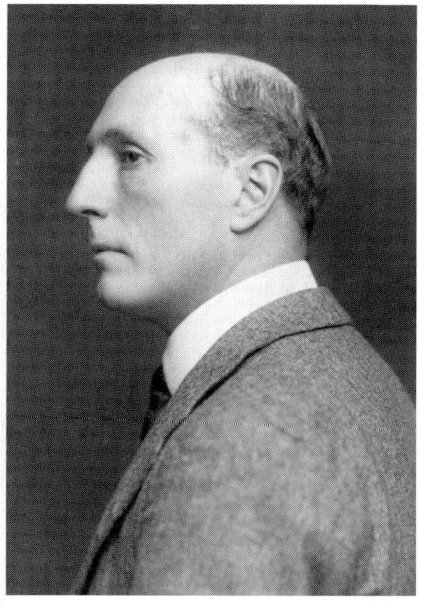

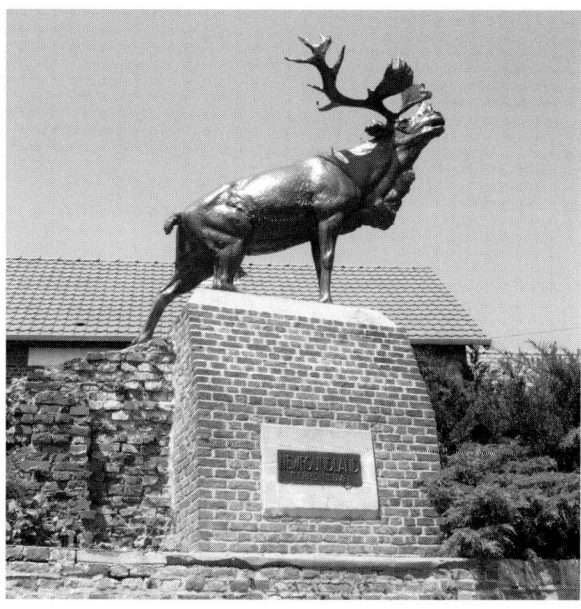

Basil Gotto. Photo: Jane Lindstrand-Gotto (Granddaughter of Basil Gotto).

Caribou war memorial monument at Monchy-le-Preux, sculpted by Basil Gotto. Reproduced by kind permission of Veterans Affairs, Canada.

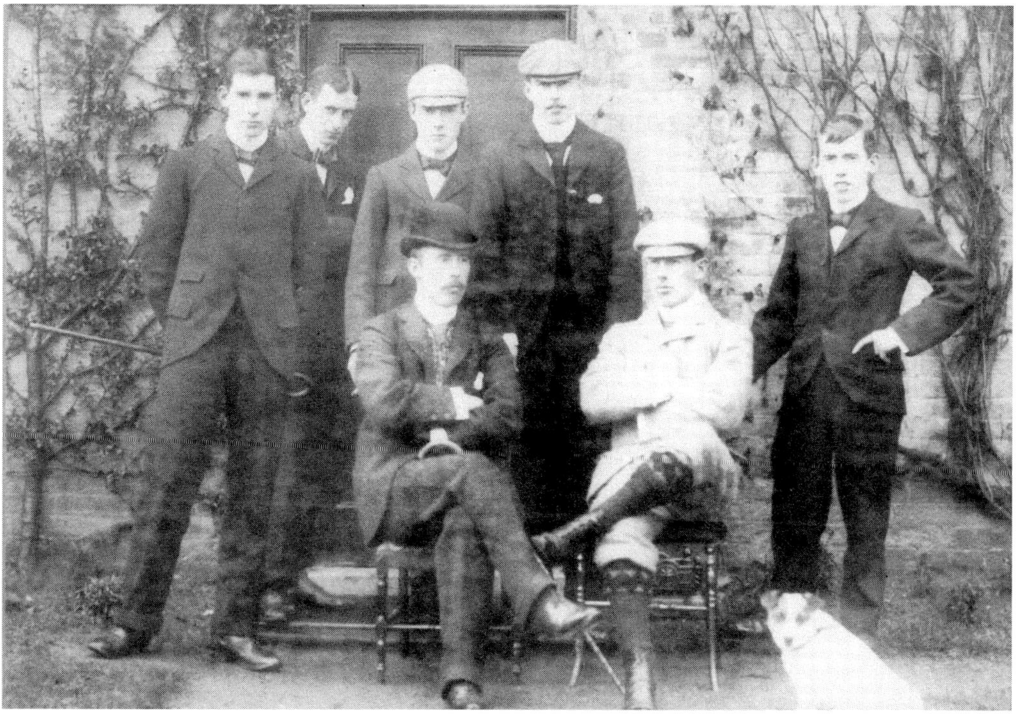

Richard King Huskinson (standing, right) at The Cottage, Epperstone, 1897, with (left to right) his brothers Edward, William, Ernest, Percy (standing), Charlie and Harold (seated). Photo: His Honour Judge Nicholas Huskinson.

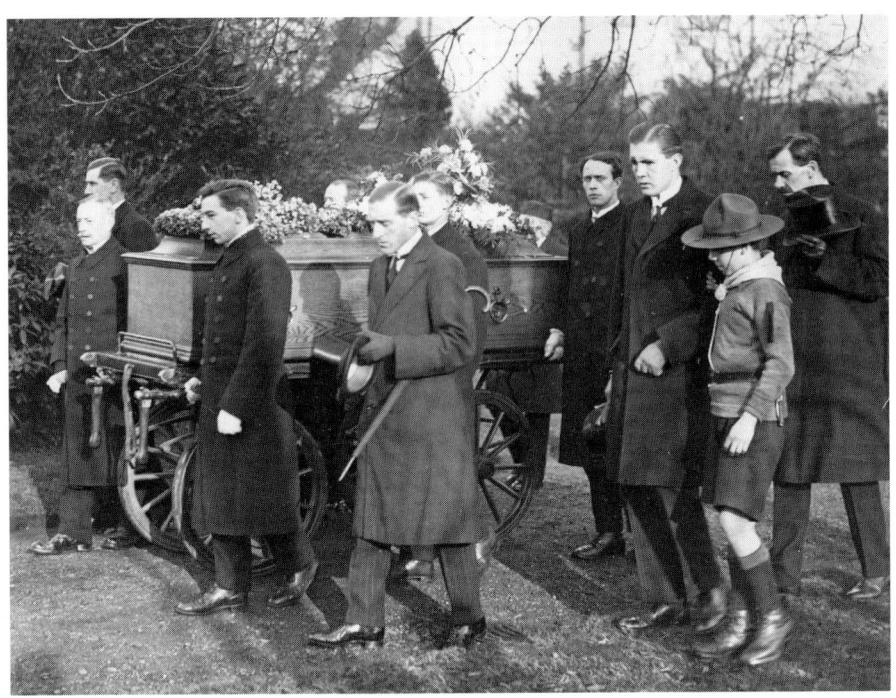

Pearson's funeral, with Ian Fraser escorted by a Scout. Photo: St Dunstan's.

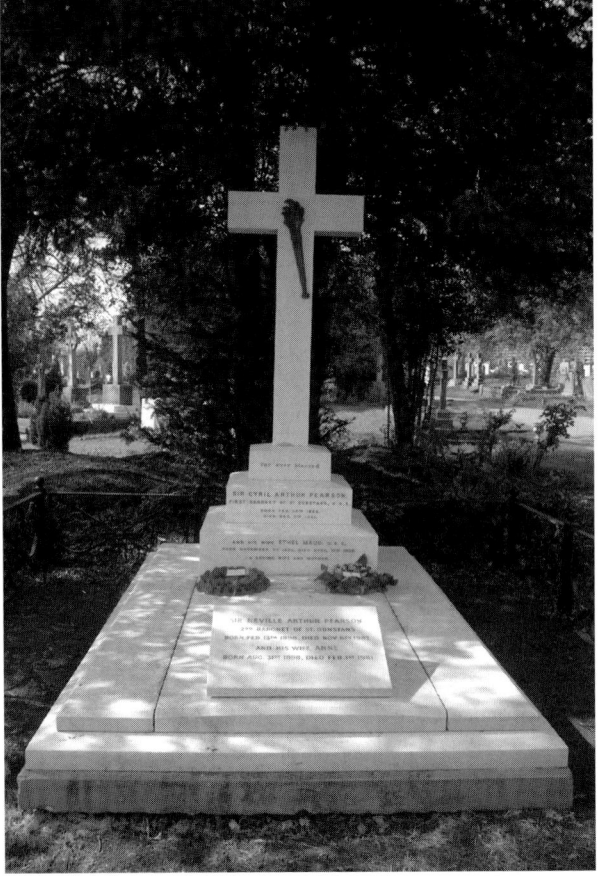

Pearson family grave, 2005. Photo: St Dunstan's.

the company of uncomprehending loved ones and friends who have no first-hand experience of warfare and with whom he can find it difficult to communicate. He quickly realises the futility of attempting to describe what he has endured (which would be a catharsis for him) and will therefore often suppress his feelings. In so doing, he feels depressed, frustrated, inadequate, and angry and can become progressively isolated.

At St Dunstan's, however, the situation is entirely different. Here, he is in the company of comrades, with whom he can relax, share a cigarette or a joke, and even discuss the war in the knowledge that he is being listened to by those who know what he is talking about. In this way, friendships are built up, both at work and at play. They face common problems, strive together to overcome them and share with each other little tips about discoveries that they have made which make life easier. Serving soldiers would also come and talk to the men if they so wished, and this sense of comradeship was the most important therapy of all.

In this new environment, acts of kindness, however small, assumed a hugely disproportionate significance. The example is given of a soldier who is sitting in the garden one day, talking to a newly arrived comrade. The comrade is complaining that his lips are painful and oversensitive – having previously been singed by the blast from a shell – to the extent that he could no longer enjoy a cigarette. 'Now don't you fret, mate', says the soldier, reaching into his pocket. 'I've got just the thing for you. I designed it myself. A tiny acorn cup holds the ciggy, like so, and then this little hollow stalk fits into the hole that I bored into the cup, like so. And there you have it – a ciggy holder!' A match is struck. The comrade feels the tiny tube between his lips. It is so tiny that he can tolerate it. He takes a deep breath. Then he coughs and splutters. 'How does that feel, mate?' asks the soldier anxiously. 'Good', replies the comrade, as he gasps for breath. 'Very good.'[18]

Consultant Ophthalmologist Sir Arnold Lawson declared that the re-education of a man becomes increasingly difficult as he grows older and more set in his ways, whereas the men of St Dunstan's, in the main, had youth on their side:

It was this spirit of youth that was the chief asset in the production of that wonderful cheeriness which so pervaded St Dunstan's during the war, and so astonished all who went there. The society of comrades severely maimed helped in a very great measure; but neither the society of comrades nor the sympathy and help of all who worked at St Dunstan's would have brought that laughter and that brightness if St Dunstan's had been peopled by old men instead of men mostly in the prime of youth.[19]

Pearson summed up the position when he referred to the

> … cheerful … active, healthy, eager, young blind men who were learning in an atmosphere of good fellowship to start life again. It is a claim which I am justified in making, that St Dunstan's is one of the most cheerful places in the kingdom.[20]

18

The Chief Visits
the Front

Pearson made two visits to France during the course of the First World War. The first was in late 1916, at the request of the King, when his purpose was to inspect 'a number of the comparatively small and scattered institutions at which the blinded French soldiers were being trained'. However, he encountered no innovations there that he thought necessary to incorporate into the St Dunstan's regime.[1] His second visit involved placing himself in jeopardy.

Pearson was aware that his blindness was actually an advantage to him in his dealings with the men, in that he knew the difficulties that they faced and understood them as no sighted person could. He was also aware, that in another respect he was at a disadvantage in that unlike them, he had no first-hand experience of the battlefields. He wondered what it was really like on the Western Front and felt that if he could experience it for himself, then he would more easily be able to empathise with the men. There was however, the problem of how could this be achieved given the intensity of the fighting, and the fact that as a blind man on the battlefield, he would be regarded as more of a liability than an asset. It was in the summer of 1917 that his wish was granted. Meanwhile, on 17 June 1917, Pearson's son Neville was commissioned as 2nd Lieutenant into the Royal Field Artillery.

In France, Pearson visited Lieutenant General Sir Henry Sinclair Horne, Commander of the British First Army (whose headquarters was at Rachincourt,

3 miles south of Bruay-la-Buissière) and took a keen interest in the 'School of Scouting, Observation, and Sniping' – the first to be established by the British Army – at Linghem in the Pas-de-Calais. The school had been created by Hesketh V. H. Prichard, who, as already mentioned, had been dispatched by Pearson in late 1900 to hunt for the giant sloth of Patagonia. Prichard had arrived at the Western Front in May 1915, at the age of 38 and with the rank of captain, as one of the officers in charge of six accredited war correspondents. For him, however, there were more urgent matters to attend to.

Prichard quickly realised the danger which German snipers posed to Allied troops: 'We lost eighteen men in a single battalion in a single day to enemy snipers.'[2] Having gained first-hand experience of the trenches, where he became a hunter of human beings, rather than of big game, Prichard persuaded Lieutenant Colonel A. G. Stuart of 40th (Pathan) Regiment, Indian Army, to procure for him the appointment of 'sniping expert' to the Third Army. The result was the establishment of the British Army's first sniping school, which offered a fourteen- to seventeen-day course in which all aspects of shooting and rifle maintenance, map and compass work, use of telescopes, fieldcraft and camouflage were covered. For his services both in the school, and in the Front Line, Prichard was awarded the Military Cross and Distinguished Service Order.

Pearson took the opportunity to pay another visit to the institutions which the French had established for their war blinded. He also discussed with the American authorities how they proposed to care for their men who might lose their sight in the conflict – the Americans having entered the war on 6 April 1917.

Pearson proceeded to Vimy Ridge, 7½ miles north-east of Arras, on a thoroughly wet day, which, he said, gave him 'a good idea of what the real thing was like on the day of the great attack'. (This was a reference to the successful storming of the Ridge by Canadian infantry, supported by the British, on 9 April of that year.) He had a special reason for choosing this particular place, for this is where his son Neville, who had served in the British Army for thirteen months, had been wounded.[3] Pearson:

> The heavy clay ground was slippery and slimy to a degree that made walking very difficult, and when one thought that on the very day the Vimy Ridge was stormed, the conditions were worse than on the day that I was there, one realised the tremendous difficulties our fellows had to overcome, and the heroism with which they overcame them.

The landscape, said Pearson was pitted with shell craters, some larger than 'a good-sized house'. He imagined that it looked 'like nothing else on earth'.

> The chalky subsoil has been churned to the top, and this upheaval of the ground could never have been brought about by any agency short of an earthquake other than the one which actually produced it. From the top of the Ridge one gets a very wide view of the surrounding country, and of the scene of operations. Batteries behind us were firing away over the Ridge, and we could see the shells crashing on the land just beyond the embankment of the railway that runs between Lens and Arras.
>
> We walked up the Ridge again from [the village of] Thelus, which was just a succession of rubble heaps, and there was very little in the way of bricks even; it was mostly dust.

Now came the moment when Pearson would experience for himself the dangers of the Western Front. He had been standing on the Ridge for two to three minutes:

> When there was a sound which I had heard before, but it seemed not quite right. Instead of the bang coming first, the 'whiz' came first. Well, it is wonderful how quickly one's head can work. It took me an extremely small percentage of a second to realise what that 'whiz' meant. The shell went over our heads and flopped down fifty yards beyond us. My guide said, 'I told you this was not a very healthy spot. We had better get into that dug out.'

Having remained in the dug out for about ten minutes, and decided that the shell was only a so-called 'searcher,' they emerged. No sooner had they done so, when another shell landed on the very spot where they had been standing when the first one had passed over their heads:

> This one was a good deal too close to be comfortable. I felt a distinct shock, and was splashed all over with mud, and I had the further experience of receiving a wound on the head from a stone. Wound is, perhaps, rather a large word, for it only took the form of a pretty sharp rap, which raised a good big bump, but it enabled me to realise just a little bit what the real thing must feel like. Six more shells followed in quick succession round us and we lost no time in getting away.[4]

Following this experience Pearson declared: 'I am convinced that I have just as clear an idea of what is going on at the Front as has anyone else who has been there lately.' This was of course an overstatement. Pearson had been at the Front for only a very short time, whereas many had served in the trenches for years. Also, his brief visit could have given him little idea of what it was like to be permanently cold, wet and hungry, to have to endure the incessant noise of bombs and shells, to see those around you being killed and maimed and being asked to take the life of another human being. Nonetheless, Pearson subsequently believed that his visit to Vimy Ridge had enabled him to forge 'another link between [himself] and his blinded soldiers'.[5] As for the men themselves, they probably had regarded his proposed visit to the Front with a mixture of incredulity and apprehension.

In March 1918, Pearson's periodical, *Pearson's Magazine* which had, up until that point opposed the War, changed its stance and decided 'to join in support of the war aims of President Wilson and the British Labour Party'.[6]

That year, Ian Fraser married Pearson's former personal assistant and guide Irene Mace. (It was she who had visited Fraser, on Pearson's behalf, at the 2nd London General Hospital, to invite him to join St Dunstan's.) In the same year, the Federation of Grocers Associations raised the money for the purchasing and equipping of West House in Brighton, which would be used by St Dunstaners who required holidays or periods of convalescence.

In May 1918, Otto Kahn, who had recently visited St Dunstan's, wrote these words to Pearson:

> What has aroused my admiration ... above all [is] the spirit of cheer, buoyancy, and courage which pervades the atmosphere of the place, and which is plainly apparent in the attitude and facial expression of the men and in the very manner of their firm and determined step.
>
> The fact that this admirable demonstration of British organising genius and practical humanity is being carried on in a house belonging to an American citizen, I like to regard as symbolic of that close and lasting and effective union between the two countries.[7]

Also in 1918, Ruby Smith, the daughter of the Head Gardener, and now aged six, showed her concern for the men by making a collection for them. This prompted the following response from Pearson:

Dear little Ruby,
The collecting box you brought me yesterday had 18s/3d in it. I think it is
very sweet of you to collect this for the blinded soldiers.
Yours sincerely,
Arthur Pearson[8]

The War ended on 11 November 1918 with the signing of the Armistice. By
this time, said Pearson, in excess of 600 St Dunstaners

> ... had already learned to be blind and had returned to their homes. Nearly
> seven hundred were still in training at St. Dunstan's and at the various annexes,
> and nearly two hundred were still in hospital [awaiting admission].

They included 70 Australians, 63 Canadians, 20 New Zealanders, and 10
South Africans. Pearson pointed out just how large the organisation which
he had founded had now become.[9] Of the personnel involved, in one way
or another, in contributing to the happiness and welfare of the men, there
were 595 women, 'including matrons; VADs; nurses; teachers of Braille,
typewriting and music; regular visitors, and those who came to read to the
men and take them for walks, and secretaries'.
The male staff of 293 made up

> ... the adjutants, the oculists, the doctors, the chaplains, the workshops'
> teachers, poultry-farm instructors, accountants, orderlies, walkers, masseurs,
> chauffeurs, porters, gardeners, scouts, and those engaged in the Pensions, the
> Settlement, and the After-Care Departments.[10]

For five and a half years, Pearson had strained every sinew to make
St Dunstan's a success, not only in the United Kingdom, but globally.
It should also be remembered that as President of the National Institute for
the Blind, this was not his only concern, for he also had connections with
homes for the blind in Chester, Bristol, Liverpool, Manchester, Bradford,
Leeds and Cardiff. In Hertfordshire, he encouraged the creation of the
Chorleywood College for Girls with little or no sight. His enthusiasm
captured the imagination of the nation, and his success at fundraising
enabled the NIB to open the 'Sunshine Home' for blind babies, also at
Chorleywood, where he demonstrated his insight into the specific problems
which they faced:

Those who are born blind, or lose their sight in infancy are at a great disadvantage, compared with others who have seen the world, and whose memories are stored with pictures of all that is in it.[11]

The result of all this hard work, said Dark, was that Pearson now suffered 'the inevitable reaction: his nerves became troublesome and his generally robust health, unsatisfactory'. The years of selfless dedication had taken their toll.[12]

During the First World War, the activities of the Fresh Air Fund had been somewhat curtailed. However, with the cessation of hostilities in 1918, the holiday season began in earnest with the traditional visit to Epping Forest. In 1919, Sir Neville Pearson was elected a member of the Fund's council, in which capacity he was in a position to help his father – for the Chief's eyesight was deteriorating to the extent that he had difficulty in reading and signing the Fund's correspondence and minutes. Sir Neville also joined his father's publishing firm C. Arthur Pearson Ltd.

19

Thomas Waldin: a St Dunstaner Goes Forth

Every St Dunstaner had his own story to tell. Nevertheless, it is illuminating to examine the life of just one of them in more detail in order to demonstrate the lengths to which Pearson was prepared to go to assist his men on an individual basis.

When, on 26 October 1916, at the Victoria Wesleyan Chapel in St John's Wood, St Dunstaner Thomas Waldin married Esther Benwell, the couple had every reason to be grateful to St Dunstan's and to the Chief. The story of Waldin, the son of Birmingham saddle tree maker (the saddle tree being the wooden frame upon which the leather saddle is constructed), is as follows.

On 20 May 1915, twelve days after his 20th birthday, Rifleman Waldin crossed the Channel from England to France with the 8th Rifle Brigade, which made its way by train and route march to Belgium's Ypres Salient. During the six months that followed, Waldin would be wounded twice and also gassed. Whilst convalescing at a farmhouse with a Belgian family he sent a postcard to his sister May. One side of it said simply: 'From Tom, Sept. 5th 1915.' On the other side was a group photograph featuring himself, together with wounded comrades who were also convalescing (some being attired in the standard issue uniform known as 'hospital blues') and his Belgian hosts. This was the last time he would put pen to paper as a sighted person.

On 30 November 1915, the 8th Rifle Brigade moved into trenches at La Brique in the north-east sector of the Salient. By now, the strength of the battalion had been reduced – by death and injury – to about 500, from its original complement of 956 officers and men.

On 4 December 1915, whilst serving on the Front Line ('firing trench'), Waldin and four of his fellow riflemen received an order which they could scarcely believe. An officer would shortly be arriving to inspect the trench and they must therefore, vacate it in order for it to be tidied up. Meanwhile, they were to clean themselves up and polish their buttons (Rifle Brigade tunic buttons being black in colour – which was unique to the British Army). The outcome was predictable. As the men stood in the open ground behind the trench, they were immediately spotted by the enemy. Two shells landed – one on either side of them – killing one and injuring four. No less than thirteen pieces of shrapnel lodged themselves in Waldin's body.

As for his eyes, the right was damaged beyond repair. It was therefore surgically excised. Embedded in the left eye was a foreign body: an elongated, nail-shaped piece of metal measuring 2¼ inches long and ¼ inch in diameter. This was surgically removed. Despite the damage which this eye had sustained, it was the opinion of the doctor that some vestige of sight might still remain in it.

Sadly, however, whilst Waldin's other wounds were being cleaned and disinfected with EUSOL (Edinburgh University Solution of Lime) by a VAD nurse who was newly arrived from England, some of the solution accidentally found its way into Waldin's left eye, causing irrevocable damage to the cornea. When Waldin learned that he would never see again, he turned his face to the wall and refused to speak for 24 hours. Further disaster struck when the hospital ship transferring him back to England was torpedoed. He was rescued but it was yet another terrifying experience for a newly-blinded man.

At the 2nd London General Hospital, Chelsea, Waldin came under the care of Major Ormond (previously mentioned as being one of St Dunstan's two consultant ophthalmologists). For the empty right eye socket, Ormond could only offer a glass replacement. For the left he would, if Waldin so wished, close it by suturing the lids together. It was shortly afterwards that Pearson came to Waldin's aid and offered him a place at St Dunstan's.

On 25 February 1916, Waldin duly arrived at St Dunstan's Lodge where shortly afterwards, he was interviewed by Pearson and told what types of training courses were on offer there. When Waldin became bewildered, having been asked to choose an occupation and not knowing how to proceed, Pearson was there to guide him. In the event, he chose boot-repairing. Pearson, however, was concerned, not only with the work-related aspects of the men's lives, but equally with their general well-being. This he would shortly demonstrate by coming to Waldin's aid in a matter concerning an affair of the heart.

It had been Matron's idea that local young ladies might like to take her St Dunstaners for walks in Regent's Park after lunch on Sunday afternoons and she consulted Pearson, who heartily concurred. For Waldin, the outcome of this was that he met a Miss Esther Benwell whose stepfather, George, was caretaker at the Victoria Wesleyan Chapel in Barrow Hill Road in nearby St John's Wood.

Having got to know one another, Esther introduced Waldin to her parents and the couple started courting. However, just as he was beginning to enjoy family life again, and in particular the company of Esther, matters came to an abrupt end. Esther's mother, Mrs Jane Benwell forbade her daughter ever to see Waldin again.

In characteristic fashion, Pearson tackled the situation head on. He arranged for the Benwells to visit St Dunstan's and meet with him in person, in order that he might ascertain what the problem was. Whereupon, Mrs Benwell told him that she had serious misgivings in respect of Waldin, in that she could not see how a blind man would possibly be able to support her daughter. (It should be noted that Esther herself had poor eyesight, and was therefore unable to work.) The Chief responded by arranging for the Benwells to have a conducted tour of the premises, where they saw the men engaged in the various training programmes which would one day enable them to support themselves.

Mrs Benwell was completely won over. Not only that, but at Pearson's invitation she joined Waldin's boot-repairing class, in order to learn how to cut out the leather templates, use the industrial treadle to sew on soles, and patch worn uppers, for no matter how well-trained a blind man may be, there are certain tasks which he simply cannot perform unaided.

Knowing that he now had the Benwells' blessing, Waldin found the courage to propose to Esther, having first asked her father's permission for his daughter's hand in marriage. She accepted.

Waldin was not the only war-blinded man to find romance at St Dunstan's, for as Pearson observed:

One very delightful feature in the record of St. Dunstan's is the number of marriages that took place. Many St. Dunstaners were of course married men, and before the end of the war more than three hundred bachelors had found wives for themselves – very delightful and charming wives as I know for I have met them all. Some of them were sweethearts of earlier days, but many romances arose, as I have already remarked, from the companionships that were formed at the dances, or during outings on the lake, or walks, or the hours of study.[1]

When Waldin completed his ten-month training period he was duly presented, as was the tradition, with his St Dunstan's Badge – with its motif of a flaming torch. This meant as much to him as any of the wartime medals which he had won.

Working premises were found for Waldin by St Dunstan's in St John's Wood, and he and Esther moved in with her parents. Six years later, in 1922, the Waldins and the Benwells decided to relocate to the city of Winchester in the southern English county of Hampshire.

When Pearson heard that Waldin was about to leave the area, he took the trouble to write him the following letter:

Dear Waldin,

I am very sorry to feel that you are leaving St. John's Wood, where you have built up for yourself so excellent a reputation as a boot-repairer.

I feel sure that you will prove yourself as successful in Winchester as you have in St. John's Wood, and I look forward to receiving enthusiastic reports of your new surroundings, and of the way in which trade is going. You are a thorough credit to St. Dunstan's, Waldin, and I am sure that you will keep the old flag flying creditably, wherever you may be. As you know my good wishes, and those of all your old friends at St. Dunstan's go with you.

With kind regards to your wife, and the best of good luck to you both,

Yours sincerely
Arthur Pearson

Chairman – Blinded Soldiers' and Sailors' Care Committee.[2]

Waldin would treasure this letter always, even though he was unable to read it. He himself wrote the following letter, which was published in the *St Dunstan's Report*:

> I thought I would write and let you know I am leaving London for Winchester. I have been in my shop at St John's Wood nearly five years and have always had great kindness shown to me by St Dunstan's. I hope that I will be able to make as big a success in my new shop as I did in the old. I owe everything I am now to Sir Arthur Pearson and St Dunstan's.

> Thomas Waldin[3]

In Winchester Waldin was visited not only by Mr Martin, St Dunstan's Aftercare Officer for the Blind, but also by C. B. Fry, who, as Director of the training ship *Mercury*, was currently living thirteen miles away at Hamble, on the south coast. As an acquaintance of Pearson from the days when he contributed articles to the *Daily Express*, Fry would undoubtedly have known about the Chief's subsequent work at St Dunstan's. Therefore, when he discovered that Waldin was in the locality, Fry took the trouble to seek him out and made a point of becoming one of Waldin's regular customers.

Despite being separated by a distance of 60 miles, St Dunstan's was never far from Waldin's thoughts. In fact, the Benwells called their house (the garage of which served as Waldin's shop premises) 'St Dunstan's', and Waldin continued to wear his St Dunstan's Badge with pride. From boot repairer, he went on to become proprietor of his own general stores, which he ran virtually single-handed – much to the astonishment of the citizens of Winchester. He and Esther raised a family of four children.

The St Dunstaners from Overseas

St Dunstaners, who came from all corners of the British Empire, were often disappointed on their return to their native lands to find that their pre-existing blind organisations were ill-prepared to take responsibility for their care. In this respect, however, the Canadians were probably better organised than most.

The Canadians

In 1916, Corporal Alexander G. Viets, who had been blinded by an exploding mortar, returned to Canada from St Dunstan's as the first war-blinded Canadian soldier to return home. Here, he resumed work with his former employees, the Imperial Life Assurance Company of Canada as a salesman.

Captain Edwin Albert Baker, MC of the Royal Canadian Engineers, a graduate in electrical engineering, was the first Canadian officer to be blinded (by a sniper's bullet). On his return home in 1916, he found employment with the Hydro Electric Power Company of Toronto (which was concerned with the harnessing of power from Niagara Falls). In

October 1916, he was recruited by the Federal Government as Consultant on Services to the War Blinded.

Together with five other Canadians, Viets and Baker founded, in 1918, the Canadian National Institute for the Blind (CNIB), of which Pearson was made Honorary President. The two men also joined the Board of Directors of Toronto's Free Library of Braille Literature, and were instrumental in expanding its facilities.

Harris Turner became a member of the Saskatchewan Legislature, where he put the debating skills which he had learned at St Dunstan's to good use. He went on to found his own newspaper, *Turner's Weekly*.[1] Private Bill Dies established his own tobacco and stationery shop. Lieutenant Thomas E. Perrett returned to Regina, provincial capital of Saskatchewan, to take up his former post as Head of the Regina Normal School Teacher Training College.

In January 1919, Pearson paid a visit to the CNIB's headquarters in Toronto. Here, he was entertained at Pearson Hall (so named in his honour) by 25 graduates of St Dunstan's, including Viets and Baker. 'We have but carried our torches from St Dunstan's, where they were lit,' declared Baker (the then CNIB Vice-President) on that occasion.[2] Pearson regretted that having visited Canada, he had not the time to pay a similar visit to Australia, New Zealand and South Africa.

The Australians

Trooper Jim 'Digger' Scrymgeour became a cattle breeder with a stud farm of 400 acres. He wrote a book entitled *The Blind Cattlemen*. Frank Marriott from Tasmania became a Member of Parliament.

When Private Charlie Hills and Lance-Corporal Elmer 'Sticky' Glew returned home, they set up an aftercare service for the returning war blinded in each Australian state. In this, they were assisted by the Australian Red Cross.

The war blinded were also cared for and trained at the Royal Victorian Institute for the Blind in Melbourne and at the Royal Blind Society in Sydney.

New Zealanders

When the first ship containing war-blinded men arrived home in 1917 (or possibly in 1918), there was literally no one in attendance, even to escort them down the gang plank to the dockside, let alone see them safely home and take responsibility for their subsequent rehabilitation and training. When this came to the notice of The Commercial Travellers' and Warehousemen's Association of New Zealand (C.T.W.A.N.Z.), it responded by setting up various branches throughout the country, in order to raise funds and assist the men – of whom there were 28 in all.[3] The Wellington War Funds Committee was also established during the First World War with its affiliated Associations of Auckland, Canterbury and Otago. From this fund, the sum of £500 was sent to St Dunstan's, London, which had done so much to help New Zealanders blinded in the conflict.

Rifleman James Chisholm, who had learnt poultry farming at St Dunstan's, became a poultry farmer on New Zealand's North Island.[4] Donald McPhee, who had been taught massage at St Dunstan's, returned home to preside over Auckland's Social Club for the Blind.[5]

Trooper Clutha Nantes Mackenzie of the Wellington Mounted Rifles (whose father Sir Thomas, was New Zealand's High Commissioner in London) was blinded at Gallipoli. He became a St Dunstaner, sharing a room with Canadians Viets and Baker. At St Dunstan's, Pearson took Mackenzie under his wing and directed his youthful energy into producing a newspaper entitled *Chronicles of the New Zealand Expeditionary Force*. Mackenzie married Doris Sawyer, a St Dunstan's VAD.

On his return home, Mackenzie helped raise funds for New Zealand's Jubilee Institute for the Blind (later the New Zealand Institute for the Blind) founded in 1891 in Parnell, Auckland, with funds raised during the celebrations for Queen Victoria's Golden Jubilee of 1887. This enabled workshops for the blind to be built in Auckland, and also a hostel – a handsome brick building with a Doric-style colonnade. It opened in 1926 and was named 'Pearson House'. Mackenzie became Director of the Jubilee Institute. In 1921, he was elected to New Zealand's parliamentary House of Representatives and was knighted in 1935. Mackenzie subsequently spent the entire period of the Second World War in India, where he established a St Dunstan's training centre for blinded Indian servicemen at Dehra Dun, 120 miles north of Delhi in the foothills of the Himalayas.[6]

South Africans

The war blinded were assisted by philanthropically-minded individuals and by the religious community, until Durban lawyer John Edward Palmer founded the Association for the Blind and started a fund for their financial assistance. It so happened that during the First World War, South Africans Charles H.Vintcent and his wife Lilian were living in London and Pearson was delighted when after the war, they offered to represent St Dunstan's in their home country on the organisation's South Africa Committee.[7]

Sergeant Walter ('Mike') Bowen returned home to study law, and he became a Member of Parliament. He went on to play an important role in creating the South African National Council for the Blind.

Indians

In India, practical difficulties that one can at least begin to imagine precluded the creation of a St Dunstan's style training establishment. However, St Dunstan's donated a lump sum to the Indian Soldiers Board, out of which 5 rupees per month was paid to every Indian blinded in the war. In 1919, St Dunstaner the Reverend W. Gilbert Speight was appointed to the post of Director of the Palmacottah School for the Blind in Southern India. His work for blind children (of all races and creeds) became so well known that similar institutions sprung up all over the subcontinent.[8]

21

Pearson and
Helen Keller

It was a series of extraordinary coincidences that brought together two of the most pre-eminent people in the world of the blind: Arthur Pearson, and American Helen Adams Keller. This began with the torpedoeing of British passenger liner *Lusitania* by a German U-Boat off the coast of Ireland on 7 May 1915. Of the 1,959 passengers and crew aboard, only 761 survived (128 Americans were lost, from a total of 197).

Travelling on the *Lusitania*, which was en route from New York to Liverpool, was George Kessler – otherwise known as the 'Champagne King' – who owned a wine importing company in New York City. Kessler also had a home in England on the banks of the Thames river at Bourne End, Hertfordshire – the same village in which Arthur Pearson had his home. For this reason it is likely that the two already knew each other.

Following the torpedoeing Kessler was thrown into the water. He managed to get into a lifeboat, but by the time he was rescued, only three of its twelve occupants remained alive. Whilst recovering in hospital in England, Kessler was visited by Pearson who told him about St Dunstan's. After his time in hospital Kessler travelled to France to be reunited with his wife Cora.

Having endured this traumatic experience, and in the light of what Pearson had told him, Kessler resolved to devote himself to helping soldiers blinded in the war. To this end, on 11 November 1915, he and Cora formally organised the British, French and Belgian Permanent Blind Relief War Fund in Paris, with French war veteran George Raverat as head of European Operations. Finally, having returned to the USA, the Kesslers enlisted the help of the legendary Helen Keller, who was then aged 35, and whose name was widely recognised around the world. Helen readily agreed to help, telling Kessler:

> My heart glows every time I think of what you are doing for the blinded soldiers. May our work grow until every man who has given his sight for his country will feel the comforting warmth of a friendly hand guiding him through a dark, strange world.[1]

Helen was born in Tuscumbia, Alabama, USA on 27 June 1880, the daughter of Captain Arthur Henley Keller – who had fought in the Confederate Army during the American Civil War – and his wife Kate Adams Keller. Tragedy quickly struck Helen, for at the age of only 19 months she became not only blind but also deaf. This is believed to have been caused either by scarlet fever or meningitis. She became increasingly aggressive, destructive and unmanageable: a classic example of someone who finds themselves being looked after by a family who, through no fault of their own, lacked the skills to help her. She also felt isolated from her peers, with whom there was no communication.

Fortunately for Helen, her mother Kate had read Charles Dickens' *American Notes for General Circulation*, (published in 1842, following that author's 5-month visit to the USA.) In it Dickens described the help and education that had been given to another blind and deaf child, Laura Bridgman of Hanover, New Hampshire by a Dr Samuel Gridley Howe. The problem was, however, that Dr Howe was now deceased.

Helen was about six years old when her father Arthur, learnt of a Dr Julian John Chisholm, an 'eminent oculist in Baltimore [Maryland] who had been successful in many cases that had seemed hopeless'.[2] Chisholm was unable to assist, but recommended to them Dr Alexander Graham Bell, inventor of the telephone, who had chosen to devote himself to the teaching of the blind. Bell, in turn, advised the Kellers to approach Michael Anagnos, Director of the Perkins Institute for the Blind in Boston, Massachusetts, where the late Dr Howe had previously worked.

The outcome was that on 3 March 1887 – shortly before her seventh birthday – Helen was introduced to the person who would transform her life: Anne Mansfield Sullivan, a former pupil of the Institute who was herself partially sighted. Anne would become Helen's tutor.

Anne began by teaching Helen to 'finger spell', whereby she would give the child an object – such as a doll – to touch, and then spell out the word 'doll' on Helen's palm with her finger. From here Helen progressed to reading; first with the aid of pieces of cardboard on which were printed raised letters and later with Braille; then to writing, both with ordinary and Braille typewriters. In May 1888, Helen duly entered the Perkins Institute where she met other blind children who were 'so happy and contented that I lost all sense of pain in the pleasure of their companionship'.[3]

In the spring of 1890, a Mrs Lamson, who had been one of Laura Bridgman's teachers, recommended that Helen consult Miss Sarah Fuller, Principal of the Horace Mann School for the Deaf, Allston, Massachusetts, so that she might be taught to speak. Miss Fuller's method of teaching was to allow Helen to touch her (teacher's) lips, and to feel their position when she made a sound. Helen would then attempt to imitate her.[4]

In October 1894, Helen progressed to the Wright-Humason School for the Deaf in New York City, 'for the purpose of obtaining the highest advantages in vocal culture and lip reading'. Sadly however, progress was in her words, 'not what my teachers and I had hoped and expected it would be', and subsequently, it was only Helen's close family and friends, who were able to understand her.[5]

From October 1896 until autumn 1900, Helen attended the Cambridge School for Young Ladies, after which she entered Radcliffe College, Cambridge, Massachusetts, where she became the first blind and deaf person ever to enroll at an institute of higher education. In June 1904, Helen graduated as Bachelor of Arts, having developed a keen interest in literature.

Helen also became an author, and it was at Radcliffe College that she met John Albert Macy who helped to edit her first book *The Story of My Life*, published in 1903. In May 1905, John and Anne (Helen's tutor) were married, whereupon Anne changed her name to Anne Sullivan Macy. The couple set up home in Wrentham, Massachusetts, and invited Helen to join them.

It was through John that Helen became a socialist. She joined the Socialist Party in 1909, and in 1913 published *Out of the Dark*, a series of essays on socialism. The following years would be spent on lecture tours in which she championed the cause of the poor, promoted rights for women, and railed against dangerous practices in the workplace – her speeches being 'translated' for the public by her faithful companion Anne.

To Helen, who was also a pacifist, the First World War was anathema. She therefore commanded the workers: 'Strike against manufacturing shrapnel and gas bombs and all other tools of murder. Be not dumb, obedient slaves in an army of destruction. Be heroes in an army of construction.'[6]

In 1918, Helen and the Macys moved to New York, and Helen began a series of fund-raising tours on behalf of the blind. In the same year, the office of the Permanent Blind Relief War Fund opened officially in Paris, and in 1919, its American branch was incorporated in New York State as the Permanent Blind Relief War Fund for Soldiers and Sailors of the Allies, with Helen Keller and Cora Kessler as members of its Board of Directors. The Fund gave financial support to St Dunstan's, UK, and also opened schools and workshops for the blind in Belgium and France.

In 1919, Helen, presumably on the strength of what she had learnt from George and Cora Kessler, visited Pearson at St Dunstan's. Sidney Dark was privy to her subsequent correspondence with Pearson, and he declared that her typewriting was quite as good as that of a sighted stenographer. In one such letter, Helen wrote to Pearson:

> You are probably tired of being told that you are the most wonderful example in the world of victory over blindness. But I should like to tell you this again. Your accomplishments will always be an incomprehensible mystery to me, though, after all, they are only the supreme proof of a point which I am never tired of making, and that is, that the greater the handicap, the greater the will and ability to surmount it, provided it is faced in the right spirit.

When Pearson sent Helen a parcel of classical novels written in Braille, she was delighted: 'I can scarcely keep my ravenous fingers off them long enough to sleep, or walk,' she declared, and compared him to the 'Three Wise Men of Versailles' (possibly a reference to one of the books that Pearson had sent her, perhaps David Lloyd George, Georges Clemenceau and Woodrow Wilson, the men would prove not to have been so wise at the Treaty of Versailles). However, whereas the wise men gave away 'mere islands, cities and valleys', Pearson, through his work for the provision of Braille books for the blind, had bestowed 'the bread of life, kingdoms of thought, and stars that shine in the darkest night! I shall only say, no one can be more grateful to another than I am to you, and shall be all my days.' The volumes sent by Pearson to Helen included works by Arnold Bennett and Sir Arthur Conan Doyle. Helen's favourites however, were those by the Russian novelists Leo Tolstoy and Ivan Turgenev.

Helen was also fulsome in her praise for other projects, apart from St Dunstan's, in which Pearson had become involved.

> All the new work you are taking up: 'houses of childhood' for sightless babies; colleges for blind girls and boys. There is something divine, universal, in the sympathy and insight with which you strive to meet every need, every aspiration of all classes of the blind.[7]

22

Basil Gotto: in Memory
of the Fallen

Six miles to the south of the southern end of Vimy Ridge, which Pearson had visited in the summer of 1917, lies the village of Monchy-le-Preux. On 14 April 1917, the Newfoundland Regiment attacked and occupied a salient to the east of the village, with the object of denying it to the Germans. The cost to the Newfoundlanders was 166 men killed, 141 wounded and 153 captured.

After the war had ended, Lieutenant Colonel the Reverend Thomas Nangle, Chaplain to the Newfoundland Regiment, approached Basil Gotto, Pearson's friend and former war correspondent at the *Daily Express*. During the First World War, Gotto had obtained the position of Staff Sergeant Musketry Instructor at Bisley, Surrey, Headquarters of the National Rifle Association. He was subsequently commissioned, and served as Staff Officer of Musketry at the Rifle Depot, Winchester, where his brief was to improve the shooting skill of, amongst other units of the Allied forces, the Newfoundland Regiment – hence his connection with the Newfoundlanders.

Nangle told Gotto that the Government of Newfoundland proposed to erect a memorial at the scene of each battle on the Western Front in which the Newfoundland Regiment had participated. Gotto's response to Nangle was as follows:'I would propose a caribou, standing on a hilltop bellowing defiance.'

The outcome was that five war memorial bronze caribous were sculpted by Gotto, and erected at Monchy-le-Preux, Beaumont Hamel, Gueudecourt, and Marcoign Masnières in France, and at Courtrai in Belgium.[1]

Other war memorials sculpted by Gotto were to the men of the Middlesex Yeomanry who fell in the Boer War (which is in the crypt of St Paul's Cathedral, London), 'The Fighting Newfoundler' and a caribou (Bowring Park, City of St John's, Newfoundland), and a memorial to the Great War in the shape of a Greek warrior sheathing his sword (which stands outside the Army and Navy Club on Pall Mall).

In 1920, Lady Pearson was made Dame Commander of the Order of The British Empire, in recognition of her work for charity. In December that year, the owner of St Dunstan's, Otto Kahn, announced that he wished to regain possession of his house. Pearson was therefore obliged to vacate the premises and relocate to St John's Lodge – another large mansion situated in Regent's Park's Inner Circle. In that year, Arsenal Football Club played a match against St Dunstan's in Regent's Park, for which members of the former team were blindfolded (apart from the goalkeeper) in order to provide a 'level playing field'.

23

Richard King Huskinson

Journalist and author Richard King Huskinson (born on 26 March 1879, and who wrote under the name Richard King) was the son of William Lambe Huskinson of Epperstone Manor, Epperstone, Nottinghamshire and his wife Emily. He was involved with St Dunstan's almost from the time of its foundation, and his association with the organisation would continue until his death in 1947.

When his brother Edward was appointed Editor of the British magazine *Tatler*, Huskinson was employed to write its book reviews. This he did under the heading, 'With Silent Friends' and his articles soon became one of the magazine's most popular features.

In his capacity as a voluntary helper at St Dunstan's, Huskinson became known as 'The Adjutant', even though he held no official rank. Otherwise, to St Dunstaners throughout the world, he became known simply as 'Mr H'. During the latter years of the First World War, he was Senior Editor of the *St Dunstan's Review*, with Ian Fraser as his assistant. In Pearson's words, Huskinson 'gave to the blinded world generally the affection, sympathy, and insight which St Dunstan's so desperately needed'.[1]

Huskinson wrote several books, including *With Silent Friends* (1917) which he subsequently dedicated to Pearson and his St Dunstaners. In it, under the heading 'How to Help the Blind', he reveals just how similar his views were to the Chief's, when, for example, he affirms how necessary it is to encourage a blind man 'to do all he can for himself' whilst at the same time remaining, 'near at hand to turn his failures into laughter and to treat his successes as a matter of course'.[2]

Huskinson's book, *Over the Fireside*, was published in 1921. As in *With Silent Friends*, the opening chapters, entitled 'Books and the Blind', 'The Blind Man's Problem' and 'How to Help', are concerned with drawing the readers' attention to the predicament of the blind. The foreword to the book is written by Pearson, who is unstinting in his praise, both for it and for its author:

> Those who buy 'Over the Fireside' will purchase for themselves the real joy of mentally absorbing the delightful thoughts which Mr. Richard King so charmingly clothes in words. And they will purchase, too, a large share of an even greater pleasure – the pleasure of giving pleasure to others – for the author tells me that he has arranged to give half of the profits arising from the sale of this book to the National Library for the Blind, thus enabling that beneficent Institution to widen and extend its sphere of usefulness.

Pearson's faith in Huskinson as an expert (albeit unqualified) in the management of the blind, is demonstrated by the fact that he entrusted the latter to write what was perhaps the most important chapter of his book, *Victory Over Blindness*. Chapter XVI is entitled 'The Psychology of the Blinded Soldier' and in it Huskinson expresses views which are exactly in accord with those of Pearson in respect of the blind man:

> His greatest need is to be treated *normally* in his abnormal circumstances ... [When he becomes depressed] ... all that is needed is care and unobtrusive kindness – the worst will pass sooner or later; there is nothing to be done *actively* until it is gone. [To perpetually remind him of the fact that he is blind] ... by stupid little tactless acts and words, should be stamped out at the very first. I am convinced that more depression of spirits is caused by the so-called 'sympathy' which he gets from the outside world and his own friends than any realisation of his misfortune. He depends upon the love and friendship which surround him for much of his happiness – as we all do.[3]

Something else which Huskinson shared with Pearson was a determination to explore other paths, aside from the one advocated by conventional Christianity; he stated that his 'one great influence' was Swiss philosopher, poet, and critic Henri Frédéric Amiel (1821–1881).[4] The are perhaps two quotations from Amiel, who became Professor of Moral Philosophy at the academy of Geneva in 1854, that are pertinent to this story.

> Learn to limit yourself, to content yourself with some definite thing, and some definite work; dare to be what you are, and learn to resign with a good grace all that you are not and to believe in your own individuality.

> The man who insists on seeing with perfect clearness before he decides, never decides.

24

Death of
the Chief

On Friday 9 December 1921, Pearson died at his home in a tragic accident. The circumstances of his death – which were revealed at the inquest – were reported extensively in *The Times* newspaper. Sir Arthur's son, Sir Neville Pearson, who since the end of the First World War had been his father's constant companion, stated that he had last seen his father alive at 11 p.m. the previous evening: 'He was in good health and spirits. He had followed his usual occupation during the day [i.e. of visiting St Dunstan's] and had been to the theatre in the evening.' (Pearson and his wife Ethel, had attended the Princes Theatre to see a performance of Gilbert and Sullivan's opera *The Yeoman of the Guard*). Continued *The Times*:

> Naomi Glennie, Head Parlourmaid, said that she called Sir Arthur at 7.15 [a.m.] and took him an early cup of tea, when he seemed as usual. 'He enquired about the weather, and said which suit he would wear. He always prepared his own bath.'

Amy Campbell, Pearson's secretary: 'He was a man who always liked to do things for himself. He was very independent and did not like people to help him.' She last saw him alive on Thursday evening. It was his custom to have breakfast at 8.30, but on Friday morning he did not come down, and after waiting for ten minutes she went upstairs to see where he was. He was not in his dressing room. She saw his body in the bath, which was full of water.

When Consultant Surgeon Sir Milsom Rees was summoned, he found Pearson

> … lying with his head under the water and face downwards. The water was discoloured with blood, and there was blood on the nozzle of the tap. There was a wound about an inch long on the right side of the forehead, which could have been caused by his falling against the tap. Death had not occurred as the direct result of the blow, but from asphyxia due to drowning.

Sir Neville described the bath, in which the water was still running, as 'enamelled' and 'rather slippery.' In fact, only the day before his father 'had mentioned that he had previously slipped in the bath'.[1]

Pearson's final conversation, said *The Times*, was with members of his household and it related to work he proposed to do on behalf of St Dunstan's in connection with a swimming tournament, which was to take place at the nearby Marylebone Swimming Baths.[2]

The Chief's insistence on being self-reliant and on refusing all help, if he could possibly avoid it, had contributed to the death of this otherwise fit and healthy man who only the previous week had been horse-riding on the South Downs.[3] Pearson had worked for the blind right up until the end; the final public duty of what Dark describes as 'his truly wonderful life' having been to open Hoole Bank Home for the Blind, Chester.

Messages of condolence were received from Their Majesties the King and Queen; Prime Minister David Lloyd George; the Mayor of St Marylebone; the Associations of South African Blinded Soldiers; New Zealand Blinded Soldiers; Australian Red Cross; Institution for Belgian War Blinded; American Permanent Blind Relief War Fund; High Commissioners of the British Dominions; innumerable institutions for the blind scattered throughout the British Empire; and from those concerned with the welfare of the blind in all parts of the world. However, as Dark pointed out: 'Deep as was the sorrow for the death of Arthur Pearson among his fellow-citizens who could see, deeper still was it among his comrades who were blind.'

The funeral service was held at the local church, Holy Trinity in Marylebone Road. The mourners included Lady Pearson, her son Neville, the three daughters of her previous marriage and nearly 1,200 blinded

St Dunstaners, past and present. (They were accommodated in a large dormitory specially erected for the purpose in the grounds of St Dunstan's, and 200 men of the Guards Brigade volunteered to act as guides for them during their stay in London.) HM Queen Alexandra, St Dunstan's Patron, sent a wreath.

Before the flower-covered coffin as it was born up the aisle walked a Boy Scout with a wreath in the form of a Union Jack, the staff of which supported a dove carrying the device, 'V.O.B.' – Sir Arthur's favourite motto, 'Victory Over Blindness'.[4]

The service was conducted by the Bishop of London the Reverend Prebendary E. N. Sharpe, and the Reverend Harold Gibb, a former St Dunstaner who had been blinded during the War. Their Majesties King George V and Queen Mary, HM Queen Alexandra (Queen Consort of the late King Edward VII), HM the Queen of Norway, and the Prince of Wales all sent representatives. George Ridding, Pearson's former headmaster from Winchester College, who was now Bishop of Southwell, was present, as was Sir Robert Baden-Powell, founder of the Boy Scout Movement. So were several cabinet ministers and high commissioners, and also high commissioners from the dominions.

Pearson was buried at Hampstead Cemetery. At his graveside, the Reverend J. A. Williams, Chaplain to St Dunstan's said a prayer, after which, led by the band of the First Grenadier Guards, the Reverend John Henry Newman's hymn, 'Lead Kindly Light' was sung:

> Lead, kindly Light, amid the encircling gloom,
> Lead Thou me on;
> The night is dark, and I am far from home,
> Lead Thou me on.
> Keep Thou my feet; I do not ask to see
> The distant scene; one step enough for me.

If ever there was a hymn appropriate for an occasion, this was it.

From the press and public alike, praise for Pearson was unstinting. *The Times*:

> He was an exceedingly active man, a fine horseman, a swimmer, and a player of the most exercising games he could find. All that he learned from his own suffering, he lavished on his fellow sufferers; and he made his private loss

the world's gain. His maxim was, 'Blindness is an opportunity.' He made St Dunstan's a household word. Newspaper proprietors gladly helped their former colleague, giving him the publicity that he needed. During the war one could hardly pick up a newspaper without finding a reference in it to St Dunstan's and its work.

The Times continued:

[Pearson] would have none of the existing practice – he said it existed – of treating them [the blind] as a God-afflicted class, whose needs were confined to religious instruction. He said … that he had received more from St Dunstan's than he had given. He himself interviewed every blind soldier repeatedly; and once, in telling a colleague of one of them [about] a boy he had travelled 60 miles to encourage, he almost broke down.[5]

The *Daily Mail*:

Sir Arthur Pearson will be remembered neither for his achievements in business nor for his unsuspected private taste in art, but for his quiet sacrifice of all ease and leisure and his own desire to help and comfort, not only the stricken soldiers, but the blind all the world over. Few men have won gratitude more enduring; none is more grievously mourned today.

The *Daily Herald*:

Ancient tradition is full of blind prophets and poets. It is an obvious and natural thing for a man whom misfortune has cheated of the outer light to turn to the inner light. Milton had his great mental vision to console him. But, however, Arthur Pearson had no such resource. He was neither prophet nor poet. He was essentially a man of the world. When he knew that his sight was going, he determined to show that a man of the world could live in the world and work in the world without eyes to see. His triumph over darkness and the wonderful way in which he carried on with the normal detail of life were the fruits of an admirable and indomitable courage.

An article by Hannen Swaffer in the *Daily Graphic* quoted Ernest Kessell, Treasurer of St Dunstan's:

If he had not been blind, he could never have brought the power and happiness into other men's lives as he did. He made his own misfortune a blessing for others, because, like the men who came to him, he himself had once seen and now was sightless. He won their confidence, always insisting that blindness was not an affliction, only a handicap.

Sir Washington Ranger, a close colleague of Pearson, who himself was blind, referred to Pearson's willpower, to the 'watchful care' which he took in matters relating to his work, which was 'the subject of amazement and admiration on the part of all who were privileged to be his colleagues' and to his 'brilliant brain and great heart'.

Finally, Ralph Blumenfeld, writing in the *Daily Express* described Pearson as 'a man of achievement, strong, vivid, a radiant figure of energy, enthusiasm and human affection … one of those rare men who are born for a purpose.'[6]

It was not only those from the world of the blind who had cause to mourn Pearson. Sir Robert Baden-Powell:

To him the Boy Scout Movement owes more than is perhaps known by the Scouts of the present day. He was, I think, the first public man to whom I spoke of the idea [of Scouting] … and his belief that there was something in it encouraged me to go ahead with it.[7]

Baden-Powell went on to describe how, thirteen years previously, Pearson had provided the Boy Scout Movement with its first office in London's Henrietta Street – with a staff of two. Now there were more than a million scouts spread all over the world. 'Sir Arthur was himself a splendid example to Boy Scouts of energy, enthusiasm, and determination', and they would mourn the loss of this great man, with his 'pluck [and] kind-heartedness … who did so much for our movement in its early days'.[8]

Pearson's obituary was published on 13 February 1922 in *The Wykehamist*, the magazine of his former school, Winchester College:

Of all Wykehamists of recent years, there is no one who has been more conspicuous in the popular eye than Cyril Arthur Pearson; there are few of whom Winchester has more reason to be proud. He used wickedly to say that he had learnt nothing at Winchester … [but] may we not venture to claim that Pearson may have learnt something of his remarkable character from his sojourn among us? ... in his Wykehamical comradeship may he not have learnt something of the joy of making other people happy, which was the main inspiration of his life?

His first thought, as soon as he could help himself, was to take an active part in helping others. His munificent gifts for the purpose of cheering dull lives have become famous. But there are scores of other instances of his generous sympathy, unknown to the public, forgotten, probably, by himself.

In regard to his time at St Dunstan's, continued the obituary:

He was himself the soul of the whole company; and he made a point of knowing closely all the 1,400 men who were trained there. A quarter of an hour with Pearson changed their whole outlook on life. 'He gave us,' says one of the St Dunstaners, 'light for darkness, courage for despair.' Wykehamists may well be proud to take their share in paying tribute to our great Wykehamist.[9]

Pearson's tombstone consists of a tall stone cross, mounted on a tiered stone plinth. It bears the simple inscription:

For ever blessed

SIR CYRIL ARTHUR PEARSON

FIRST BARONET OF ST DUNSTAN'S C.B.E.

On the vertical arm of the cross is depicted a flaming torch – the emblem of St Dunstan's.

25

Aftermath:
Pearson's Legacy

It would perhaps have amused Pearson to know that his death provided yet another fundraising opportunity, in the shape of The Sir Arthur Pearson Memorial Fund, which was launched at the suggestion of his widow Lady Pearson. The proceeds of this fund would be divided equally between St Dunstan's ('for the care and after-care of soldiers and sailors blinded in the war, of whom there were about 2,000 throughout the Empire'), the NIB and other Empire charities for the blind. Firstly, however, 2½ per cent of the net proceeds were to be donated to the Fresh Air Fund for children, the first charity in which Pearson had become involved.[1]

Despite the tragic and untimely loss of its creator and leading light, St Dunstan's lived on. St Dunstaner Ian Fraser, the able, young former army officer whom Pearson had placed in charge of the Aftercare Department, succeeded Pearson as Chairman at the age of 24. The widowed Lady Pearson became St Dunstan's first President: a post which she held until 1947, when she was succeeded by her son Sir Neville, who held this office until 1977.

Pearson's son, Sir Neville, was appointed President of the Fresh Air Fund and Lady Pearson became a Trustee and Member of its Council. Lady Pearson also served from 1922 until her death in 1959 at the age of 89, as Vice President of the RNIB. As for the Fresh Air Fund, Sir Neville replaced his late father as its President on 18 January 1922.

In 1922, when ophthalmologist Sir Arnold Lawson, in accordance with the Pearsons' wishes, published his book *War Blindness at St Dunstans*, he paid this tribute to the Chief in the book's preface:

> I offer this result of my endeavour to the illustrious memory of the Great Founder of St Dunstan's, a man whose life was given to others, that they, like he, should see light in darkness.

For many years following the end of the First World War, men continued to present themselves at St Dunstan's with the long-term complications of eye damage sustained in that conflict. This was the case even as late as the 1950s and 1960s.

During the course of the Second World War, which ended in May 1945, just over 1,000 war-blinded had come to St Dunstan's, of whom, according to Fraser:

> ... over 300 had regained a useful degree of vision, and 100 had transferred to other institutions after treatment at our hospital. The remaining 600 would be St Dunstaners for the rest of their lives.[2]

Fraser also anticipated correctly (from the experience of the First World War) that men and women with long-term complications of wartime eye injuries would continue to be admitted to St Dunstan's for many years to come.

In the 20th century, St Dunstan's cared not only for ex-service men and women who had been blinded in two world wars, but also in other conflicts in such places as Palestine, Korea, Suez, East Africa, Malaya, Borneo, Aden, Cyprus, Northern Ireland, the Falkland Islands and the Middle East.

Pearson's other great legacy was of course the *Daily Express* newspaper, which also continues to flourish. Not only that, its current proprietor Richard Desmond is passionately concerned with the welfare of the blind. To this end, he donated the sum of £2.5 million to London's Moorfields Eye Hospital NHS Foundation Trust. The result was the Richard Desmond Children's Eye Centre which was opened by HM The Queen on 23 February 2007. Sir Thomas Boyd-Carpenter, the hospital's Chairman said: 'Moorfields includes the largest concentration of ophthalmologists anywhere in the world. Children represent a very important part of our work.'

Epilogue

Arthur Pearson lived two lives: the first in the world of the sighted; the second in the world of the blind. In the first life he was a person of considerable achievement – educating and entertaining the nation with his newspapers and publishing empire. Continuing from his first life into his life was his love of nature and the countryside, his enjoyment of horse-riding, and above all his humanity, compassion and great sense of social obligation.

One may visualise him as a schoolboy at Winchester College: sociable, witty, popular; a good 'all-rounder'. Yet here, he was hit by a double misfortune: that of having to leave school prematurely, due to the impecuniousness of his father, and of having to confront the fact that his eyesight was beginning to fail.

Nonetheless, by applying himself diligently, and by bringing his undoubted charm and talents to bear to persuade others to back him, he succeeded in founding his own publishing house.

In an appreciation of his late father, which he wrote in 1958 for the Scout Movement, Sir Neville Pearson described not only 'the spirit of gaiety and adventure' of both his father and Baden-Powell, but also the 'understanding of the young which filled the minds and hearts of these two men'. This, of course, is what led Pearson to create his Fresh Air Fund, and to give his invaluable support to Baden-Powell's Scout Movement. And it was this gaiety, sense of adventure, and understanding, that Pearson brought to the lives of his own children, as his son Sir Neville's appreciation indicates:

Primarily, he was a very lovable man, and one who made things around him into things which he intensely enjoyed. I think that he never lent his energies to anything into which he could not also throw his whole heart and being ... Those who came to stay with him were infected by his spirit of getting out of life all the fun which it could provide.

For example, Pearson used to enjoy tennis matches, as this article published in the *New York Times* indicates:

That it is possible for a blind man to follow a lawn tennis match intelligently was demonstrated by Sir Arthur Pearson ... [who] had a sound knowledge of tennis before his affliction [not a word which Pearson would have chosen himself!] came upon him. It is recorded that when a spectator of a match in which his son was participating at the Beau Sits Courts in Cannes, he was able to follow the progress of the rallies and indicate the character of the play. He did this, not by listening to comments of his neighbours, but by attending to the movements of the players' feet on the hard surface and drawing deductions which were rarely at fault.[1]

Speaking of the Pearson family home, Frensham Place, Sir Neville recalls with affection the

... small plantations of fir trees in which we children, in the spirit of Red Indians, loved to camp, and which we were prepared to defend at all costs and against all-comers. One hot summer day, lying at the edge of our plantation, we suddenly spied across the valley a hoard of the 'enemy', led by 'B-P' and my father, climbing over the iron fence and advancing with great determination towards our stockade. Of course, everyone enjoyed the ensuing battle tremendously [between] the Red Indians on the one hand, and the 'great soldier' covered with the glories of Mafeking and the South Africa Campaign, and a newspaper man who was then trying to struggle with nine daily papers and a sheaf of periodicals on the other.[2]

Pearson must have hoped, desperately, that the eye operation which he underwent in March 1908 would bring about some amelioration of his condition, if not a complete cure. Sadly, it was not to be and from that time onwards he was neither able to read nor to write. Six years later, in 1914, he became completely blind, and two years after that he relinquished ownership of the *Daily Express* newspaper. By then, his life had taken a completely different course.

In assessing the contribution made by Pearson to the world of the blind, it is pertinent to ask, what would have been the fate of the blinded soldiers, sailors, and airmen from the British Empire who came to St Dunstan's as a result of the First World War, had there been no such organisation to assist them? The answer is an unhappy one, for, as already mentioned, they would have been sent straight home from hospital to eke out a meagre existence on a pitifully inadequate pension, supplied by a parsimonious and uncaring government; to dwell amongst well-meaning relatives and friends, who would often look after them inappropriately.

Pearson had taken an interest in the blind even before he founded St Dunstan's with his work for the NIB. And even prior to that, he had conquered his own blindness. As his son Sir Neville remarked when his father became blind in 1914, he was 'unable to distinguish light from darkness'.[3] Despite this, Pearson was undeterred. In fact, so determined was he to achieve 'Victory Over Blindness', that some might say he was in denial of his own condition. Neville:

> He would have his blind men talked to of things seen, so that they could make mental pictures of them. When taking his escort – he did the taking – for a walk near Bourne End [where his home was], he would stop to point out this laburnum tree or that prospect over the river. He refused to recognise his own disability.[4]

Pearson reacted positively. He used the fact of his own blindness to good effect, by seeing himself as being in a unique position to assist the war-blinded men. He also felt a strong sense of obligation towards them on account of the sacrifice that they had made. This is evident in the foreword to his book *Victory Over Blindness* in which he dedicates the volume not only to his immediate colleagues, but to the

> … innumerable kindly and sympathetic folk [who] have helped in a thousand ways to make the men at St Dunstan's happy, to repay, as best might be done, the debt which is owed to them.[5]

And again, in the final chapter of *Victory over Blindness*, he declares:

> All that was done at St Dunstan's was a tribute to the soldiers blinded in the
> war, some recognition of what was owed to them, the most practical form of
> sympathy that could be offered, an expression of gratitude.[6]

Rifleman Thomas Waldin is cited as an example of what Pearson achieved
in the case of just one man. Pearson first met Waldin in early 1916, when the
latter was in the depths of despair, having just been informed that he would
never see again.

By contrast, this is an excerpt from a letter, which Waldin wrote – or
rather, which his daughter Jean wrote, to his dictation – to his son Peter
twenty years later. It exudes happiness: that of a contented family man with
a loving wife, who is gainfully employed, and who has many friends and
interests. He wrote:

> I am depending on a knock-kneed girl [Jean] to write for me. I have
> been doing a lot of walking lately, accompanying Jean on her egg-buying
> expeditions [she had decided to try her hand at purchasing hens' eggs and
> selling them for a profit], and everyone tells me how well I look. When Jean
> and I walk to the very top of Stanmore Lane, she walks as if her legs won't
> carry her and I walk like a two year old and it's no trouble. I'm getting much
> fatter, especially round the corporation [waist] so I hope by the time you
> come home you won't mistake me for 'Fatty Arbuckle' [the American silent
> film comedian who died in 1933].[7]

Hundreds of other St Dunstaner's would have their own unique stories
to tell.

Was Pearson, whose father and grandfather were Church of England
clergyman and whose family motto was, 'In Deo Spes' – 'In God is my
Hope', a Christian himself? As already mentioned, there are very few
references to Christianity in his book *Victory Over Blindness*. However, there
is one very significant statement in it, where he refers to a seat situated
under the mulberry tree on the lawn at St Dunstan's: 'If you look on the
back of the seat as you rise from it, you will see these words are written,' and
he quoted the following lines:

The kiss of the sun for pardon,
The song of the birds for mirth,
You're nearer to God in a garden
Than anywhere else on Earth.

On 15 May 1915, a poem about the blind by English poet, Edmund Gosse, was published in *The Blinded Soldiers and Sailors Gift Book*.[8] In it, God is asked:

Who are these luckless men
Who stumble in the gloom …
[Who] climb with faltering steps
The staircase of the night,
And see no star of Thine?

To which God replies, reassuringly:

Yet am I always with them in the darkness still
I calm then with a beam of secret light divine;
Their spirits, like an emptied cup, My hands re-fill
With purer, stronger wine.

Before He finally offers them hope:

My servant, memory, comes to paint at My behest
The walls of that dark cell which is their
teeming brain
With blowing trees, a rose, a sunset in the west,
Blue moorlands after rain.

Pearson treated his men in a holistic way: 'the treating of the whole person including mental and social factors, rather than just the symptoms of a disease'.[9] In so doing, he changed the attitude of the general public completely, not only towards his St Dunstaners, but also towards blind people in general.

The wreath, sent by HM Queen Alexandra on the occasion of Pearson's funeral, summarised the Chief's life most appositely and succinctly:

Life's race well run,
Life's work well done,
Life's crown well won.
Now comes rest.

From Alexandra.

Appendix A: Chronology of Events
at St Dunstan's

1923   The organisation was incorporated under the Companies Act, whereupon its name became official.

1925   St Dunstan's' patron, HM Queen Alexandra died. She was succeeded by HM King Edward VIII, HM King George VI, and finally, HM Queen Elizabeth II.

1932   Pearson's son Sir Neville, became Honorary Treasurer.

1923   St Dunstan's received a visit from HM King George VI.

1934   Ian Fraser was knighted.

St Dunstan's, together with the NIB, produced the first 'talking book' – in the form of a gramophone record. It also established, with the generous help of motor car magnate and philanthropist Lord Nuffield, a library of such items for the use of the blind.

1938   A new, six-storey building in the art deco-style, was completed at Ovingdean near Brighton. This would serve St Dunstan's as a holiday and convalescent home and training centre.

1939–1945, Second World War
The outbreak of the Second World War in September 1939, found St Dunstan's well prepared: St Dunstan's Ovingdean having built a new hospital wing. This housed a modern operating theatre, which was funded by Lord Nuffield.

1940 St Dunstan's was obliged to move away from the south coast as it was considered too dangerous to remain there. It established a wartime training centre at Church Stretton in Shropshire. In September 1940, a bomb fell on St Dunstan's headquarters in the grounds of St John's Lodge, destroying the talking book studios and workshop. The headquarters was subsequently re-established in nearby Park Crescent.

1941 HRH The Princess Royal visited St Dunstan's.

1942 By the end of the year, as a result of the training which they received at the machine shop at Church Stretton, over 100 St Dunstaners were at work in factories using lathes, presses, routers and upholstery equipment. By now, the first of the wartime female St Dunstaners had been admitted.

1943 A research department was set up to devise aids for St Dunstaners who had lost both their sight and their hands.

1945 St Dunstan's admitted the youngest person ever: a 13-year-old boy, blinded whilst on manoeuvres with the Air Training Corps.

1946 St Dunstaners numbered 1,673 from the First World War and 686 from the Second World War.

Many prisoners of war returning from the Far East had endured deprivation, cruelty and forced labour at the hands of the Japanese. Of these, some had become blind through injury, others from the effects of malnutrition and beriberi (deficiency of vitamin B1 – thiamine.) Because this disease frequently caused neurological damage, sufferers had the added disadvantage of being unable to read Braille – having lost sensation in their fingers.

St Dunstan's left Church Stretton and returned to Ovingdean.

British war leader Sir Winston Churchill attended St Dunstan's New Year Dance, where he presented Sir Ian Fraser with a new walking stick to commemorate his having served for 25 years as Chairman.

Sir Ian had lost his previous stick in 1944 in the Blitz, when his house had been destroyed by enemy bombing.

A new headquarters for St Dunstan's was established at 191 Marylebone Road, London.

1948   In February, HM Queen Elizabeth the Queen Mother paid her first visit to St Dunstan's, Ovingdean.

1957   West House was renamed Pearson House in honour of Sir Arthur.

1958   Ian Fraser was made a life peer.

1959   Lady Pearson died on 10 April 1959 in her 90th year. By that year, St Dunstan's had catered for over 5,000 blinded servicemen of whom 2,500 still survived, including 1,300 from the First World War and 1,200 from the Second World War and after. Of these, 550 were living overseas in establishments affiliated to St Dunstan's.

1962   In July 1962, HM The Queen and HRH The Duke of Edinburgh visited Ovingdean.

1965   Continuing the Pearson family's association with St Dunstan's, Nigel, son of Sir Neville Pearson, became a Member of its Council.

1971   St Dunstan's Ovingdean was renamed Ian Fraser House in honour of the late Chairman.

1972   Pearson House was rebuilt to provide residential accommodation and in a new wing there were facilities for the permanent nursing or convalescence of St Dunstaners following illnesses or operations.

1974   Lord Fraser died, having served as Chairman of St Dunstan's for 53 years. He was succeeded by Ion Garnett-Orme.

1976   The Chief's grandson and Council Member Nigel Pearson died.

1977   Sir Neville Pearson resigned from the presidency of St Dunstan's.

1978   Lady Fraser died. She is buried with her husband; the depiction on their joint tombstone describing her as, 'A LOVING WIFE AND MOTHER'.

1982   Sir Neville Pearson died. He is buried with his parents, as is his wife Anne who had died in the previous year.

1983   Garnett-Orme retired and Admiral of the Fleet Sir Henry Leach, GCB, DL, became Chairman of St Dunstan's.

1984   St Dunstan's moved its headquarters to 12–14 Harcourt Street, London.

1985   HM The Queen visited Ovingdean and formally opened the new South Wing, which would be used specifically to accommodate St Dunstaners and their spouses.

1990   On 1 August, HM The Queen gave permission for a garden party to be held at Buckingham Palace to celebrate the 75th Anniversary of St Dunstan's. The finale was provided by Dame Vera Lynn who sang wartime songs, including: 'We'll Meet Again'.

1991   Three servicemen were admitted as a result of the Gulf War.

1995   Pearson House was sold.

Ian Fraser House reverted to its original name of St Dunstan's Ovingdean.

1996   A post-war St Dunstaner became the first blind person to reach the summit of the highest mountain in the Alps: Mont Blanc via the First Classic Ascent Route.

1998   Ovingdean was visited by HRH The Duke of York.

2000   St Dunstan's amended its constitution to provide support for ex-servicemen and women whose visual loss met the organisation's criteria, whatever the cause of their blindness.

2001 On 15 May, HM The Queen and HRH The Duke of Edinburgh attended a reception at Buckingham Palace to commemorate St Dunstan's 85th Anniversary (in 2000).

A 14-year-old Army cadet, who had been blinded by a booby-trapped torch, joined St Dunstan's.

2003 In October, HRH The Duke of Kent visited Ovingdean.

2004 St Dunstaner Ray Hazan, a Captain in the Royal Anglian Regiment, who was blinded and lost his right hand and a considerable amount of his hearing in 1973, was elected President of St Dunstan's.

2005 Three post-war St Dunstaners were made Freemen of the City of London on 13 October. The ceremony took place at the Mansion House.

A new St Dunstan's residential training centre was opened in Sheffield.

St Dunstan's Today

St Dunstan's, the national charity continues to provide crucial assistance to blind ex-servicemen and women and their families. St Dunstaners are offered lifelong support which enables them to regain their independence, meet new challenges and achieve a better quality of life.

The Royal National Institute for the Blind

To this day, the Pearson Staff Memorial Benefit Fund seeks to alleviate need amongst RNIB staff and former staff members.

The Fresh Air Fund

Launched by Pearson in 1892, The Fresh Air Fund's name was changed in 1981 to 'Pearson's Holiday Fund'. With HM The Queen as its patron, it is still helping poor, needy, and disadvantaged children to enjoy a holiday in Britain.

The *Daily Express*

Continues to this day as a successful newspaper.

Appendix B: Pearson Family Tree

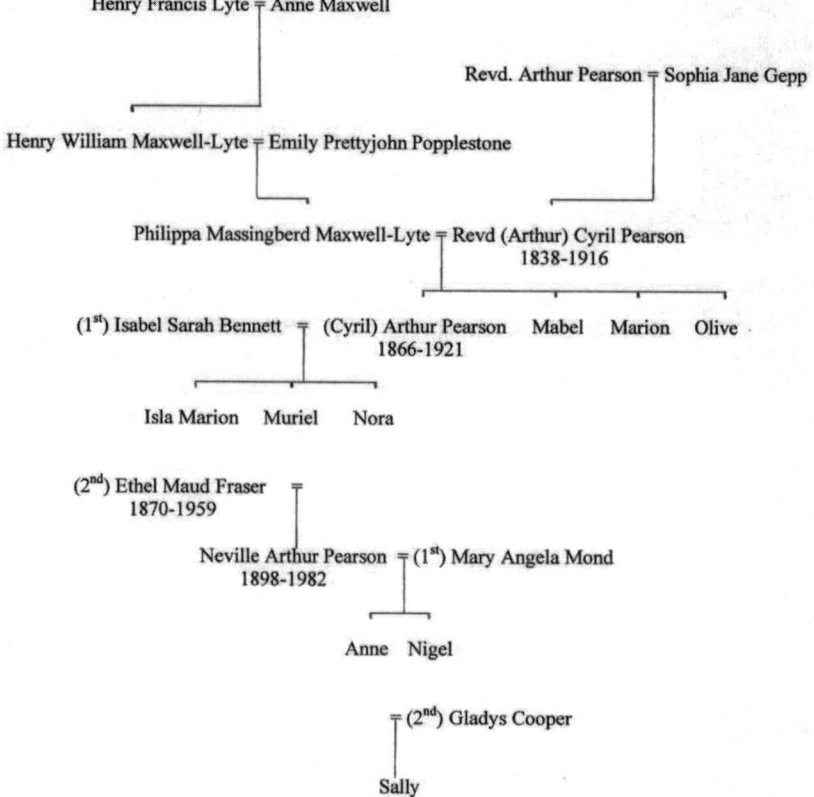

Henry Francis Lyte = Anne Maxwell

Revd. Arthur Pearson = Sophia Jane Gepp

Henry William Maxwell-Lyte = Emily Prettyjohn Popplestone

Philippa Massingberd Maxwell-Lyte = Revd (Arthur) Cyril Pearson
1838-1916

(1st) Isabel Sarah Bennett = (Cyril) Arthur Pearson   Mabel   Marion   Olive
1866-1921

Isla Marion   Muriel   Nora

(2nd) Ethel Maud Fraser =
1870-1959

Neville Arthur Pearson = (1st) Mary Angela Mond
1898-1982

Anne   Nigel

= (2nd) Gladys Cooper

Sally

Notes

Chapter 1: Arthur Pearson: Early Life
1. Obituary, Cyril Arthur Pearson, *The Wykehamist*, 13 February 1922.
2. Ibid.
3. Ibid.
4. Dark, Sidney. *The Life of Sir Arthur Pearson*, p.26.
5. Ibid.
6. Ibid.
7. 'Rats', by Arthur Pearson, *The Cornhill Magazine*, May 1899.
8. Dark, op.cit., p.42.

Chapter 2: *Pearson's Weekly*: Pearson's Magazine
1. Sir Neville Pearson, 1958. Article written about his late father for the Scout Movement, in Heasman, pp.42–3.
2. *St Dunstan's Review*, in Heasman, p.11.

Chapter 3: Pearson's Fresh Air Fund
1. Heasman, Robert. *Who was Cyril Arthur Pearson?* pp.38–9.
2. Ibid, pp.3, 39.
3. Ibid, pp.21, 22.
4. Ibid, pp.21, 22, 24.
5. Ibid, pp.24–5.

Chapter 4: Pearson Remarries: Frensham Place
1. *St Dunstan's Review*, in Heasman, p.11.
2. *This England*, in Heasman, p.12.
3. Dark, Sidney. *The Life of Sir Arthur Pearson*, p.7.
4. Gotto, Basil. *Memoir*, p.155.
5. Dark, op.cit., p.20.
6. *St Dunstan's Review*, in Heasman, p.11.

Chapter 6: Pearson the Newspaper Proprietor: Tariff Reform
1. Parker, Eric. *Hesketh Prichard*, pp.45–6.
2. *St Dunstan's Review*, in Heasman, p.11.
3. Fry, C. B. *Life Worth Living*, p.176.
4. Gotto, Basil. *Memoir*, pp.151, 152.

Chapter 7: Pearson and the Search for the Giant Sloth
1. Prichard, Hesketh V. H. *Through the Heart of Patagonia*, p.xii.
2. Menzies, Gavin. *1421: The Year China Discovered the World*. pp.270–72.
3. Piri Reis map, Note XXIII, in McIntosh, G. C. *The Piri Reis Map of 1513*. p.44.
4. Ibid, Note XXIV.
5. Darwin, Charles. *The Origin of Species*, p.334.
6. Prichard, op.cit., Appendix A, I.
7. Ibid, Appendix A, III.
8. Ibid, p.xiii.
9. Ibid, Appendix A, IV.
10. Ibid, Appendix B.
11. Parker, Eric. *Hesketh Prichard*, p.65.
12. Ibid, Appendix A, IV.
13. Parker, op.cit., p.67.

Chapter 8: C. Arthur Pearson Ltd: Pearson the Author: Pearson and the Occult
1. Dark, Sidney. *The Life of Sir Arthur Pearson*, p.8.
2. The Concise Oxford Dictionary.
3. Dark, op.cit., p.22.
4. Gotto, Basil. *Memoir*, pp.155, 156.

Chapter 9: Pearson and the Scout Movement
1. Everett, Sir Percy. *The First Ten Years*, p.7.
2. Ibid, p.8.
3. Ibid, p.8.
4. Baden-Powell, Robert S. S. 'The Late Sir Arthur Pearson', published in *Headquarters Gazette*, January 1922.
5. Dark, Sidney. *The Life of Sir Arthur Pearson*, p.21.
6. Everett, op.cit., p.8.
7. Baden-Powell, Robert S. S. *Scouting for Boys*, Appendix.
8. Everett, op.cit., p.11.
9. Baden-Powell, Robert S. S. *Scouting for Boys*, Appendix.
10. Pearson to Hesketh V. H. Prichard, 26 May 1912, in Eric Parkers's *Hesketh Prichard*, p.120.

Chapter 10: Pearson and the National Institute for the Blind
1. Dark, Sidney. *The Life of Sir Arthur Pearson*, p.218.
2. Ibid, p.143.
3. Fraser, Lord, of Lonsdale. *My Story of St Dunstan's*, p.35.
4. Dark, op.cit., pp.144-45.
6. Pearson, Sir Arthur. *Victory Over Blindness*, p.13.
7. Fry, C. B. *Life Worth Living*. P.176.

Chapter 11: Pearson and the Founding of St Dunstan's
1. Pearson, Sir Arthur. *Victory Over Blindness*, pp.57, 58.
2. Ibid, p.12.
3. Ibid, p.25.
4. Ibid, p.11.
5. Pearson, op.cit., p.38.
6. *Saint Dunstan's Annual*. 1935. London: S.C.S., 5 Gower Street. Article entitled 'Clock of 1671 to Return.' (In the year 1935, when Viscount Rothermere purchased St Dunstan's Lodge, he decided to return the clock to its original owners, the Church of St Dunstan-in-the-West.)

Chapter 12: The Newcomer to St Dunstan's
1. Lawson, Sir Arnold. *War Blindness at St Dunstan's*, p.129.
2. Pearson, Sir Arthur. *Victory Over Blindness*, pp.68–70.
3. Ibid, pp.35–6.
4. Dark, Sidney. *The Life of Sir Arthur Pearson*, p.166.
5. Fraser, Lord, of Lonsdale. *My Story of St Dunstan's*, p.37.
6. Castleton, D. *Blind Man's Vision*, p.21, and St Dunstan's: *A Story of Accomplishment*, p.2.

Chapter 13: Types of Eye Injury Sustained and Treatment
1. Pearson, Sir Arthur. *Victory Over Blindness*, pp.319, 320.
2. Lawson, Sir Arnold. *War Blindness at St Dunstan's*, p.136.
3. Ibid, p.35.
4. Ibid, pp.36, 38, 41.
5. Article 23 of The Hague Convention IV of 18 October 1907 (a convention respecting the laws and customs of war on land) came into force on 26 January 1910. Signed by virtually all the major European powers, it declared that, 'It is especially forbidden … to employ poison or poisoned weapons.'
6. *The Saint Dunstan's Annual*. 1935. London: S.C.S., Gower Street. Article entitled 'The St Dunstan's Institute' by Greville Robins.
7. Lawson, op.cit., p.47.
8. Dark, Sidney. *The Life of Sir Arthur Pearson*, p.159.

Chapter 14: Pearson's Brainchild in Operation

1. Pearson, Sir Arthur. *Victory Over Blindness*, pp.120, 121.
2. Fraser, Lord, of Lonsdale. *My Story of St Dunstan's*, p.116.
3. Pearson, op.cit., pp.125–26.
4. Ibid, p.123.
5. Ibid, p.136.
6. Fraser, op. cit., p.134.
7. Pearson, op.cit., pp.151, 152, 46, 47.
8. Ibid, pp.166, 167.
9. Pearson, op.cit., p.43.
10. Ibid, pp.168, 169.
11. Fraser, op.cit., p.46.
12. *The Times*, 21 January 1947. Sir Arnold Lawson's Obituary.
13. Fraser, op.cit., pp.74–6.
14. Ibid, p.117.
15. Obituary, Cyril Arthur Pearson, *The Wykehamist*, 13 February 1922.
16. Pearson, op.cit., p.48–9.
17. Ibid, p.193.
18. Dark. op.cit., pp.164–5.
19. Pearson, op.cit., p.205–7.
20. Fraser, op.cit., p.166.
21. Ibid, p.160.
22. Pearson, op.cit., p.167.
23. Ibid, p.317.
24. Ibid, p.280, 281.
25. Dark, op.cit., p.168.
26. Pearson, op.cit., p.299.

Chapter 15: A Successful St Dunstan's: Aftercare

1. Fraser, Lord, of Lonsdale. *My Story of St Dunstan's*, p.36.
2. Pearson, Sir Arthur. *Victory Over Blindness*, p.23.
3. Ibid, p.20.
4. Ibid, p.50.
5. Dark, Sidney. *The Life of Sir Arthur Pearson*, p.139.
6. Ibid, p.16.
7. Fraser, p.53.
8. Dark, op.cit., pp.173–74.
9. Ibid, pp.183–191.
10. *St Dunstan's Annual Report* for year ending March 1920.
11. Ibid, p.180–81.

Chapter 16: Gladys Cooper, the Fresh Air Fund and St Dunstan's
1. Cooper, Gladys. 1931. *Gladys Cooper*, pp.19, 28.
2. Ibid, p.67.
3. Ibid, p.85.
4. Ibid, p.152.
5. Ibid, p.157.
6. Ibid, pp.157–8.
7. Ibid, p.158.

Chapter 17: Pearson's Winning Formula
1. Fraser, Lord, of Lonsdale. *My Story of St Dunstan's*, pp.67–8.
2. Pearson, Sir Arthur. *Victory Over Blindness*, pp.296–97.
3. Ibid, p.118.
4. Ibid, pp.60–1.
5. Ibid, p.318.
6. Ibid, p.319.
7. Fraser, op.cit., p.169.
8. Pearson, op.cit., pp.13, 14.
9. Fraser, op.cit., pp.116–18.
10. Pearson, op.cit., p.14.
11. Fraser, op.cit., p.55.
12. Pearson, op.cit., p.52.
13. Ibid, pp.55, 56.
14. Fraser, op.cit., p.54.
15. Lawson, Sir Arnold. *War Blindness at St Dunstan's*, p.111.
16. Fraser, op.cit., p.68.
17. Ibid, p.70.
18. Information supplied by Jean Norman (née Waldin.)
19. Lawson, op.cit., p.130.
20. Dark, Sidney. *The Life of Sir Arthur Pearson*, p.159.

Chapter 18: The Chief visits the Front
1. Pearson, Sir Arthur. *Victory Over Blindness*, p.27.
2. Prichard, Hesketh V. H. *Sniping in France*.
3. *New York Times*, 16 February 1922.
4. Prichard, op.cit., pp.110–14.
5. Dark, Sidney. *The Life of Sir Arthur Pearson*, p.176.
6. *New York Times*, 21 March 1918.
7. *The Times*. A Symbol of Union. 27 May 1918.
8. Castleton, D. *Blind Man's Vision*, pp.21–22.
9. Dark, op.cit., p.176.

10. Pearson, op.cit., pp.31–2.
11. Ibid, p.14.
12. Dark, op.cit., p.201.

Chapter 19: Thomas Waldin: A St Dunstaner Goes Forth
1. Pearson, Sir Arthur. *Victory Over Blindness*, p.297.
2. Sir Arthur Pearson to Thomas Waldin, Wednesday 16 November 1921.
3. *St Dunstan's Report*, year ending 31 March 1922.

Chapter 20: The St Dunstaners from Overseas
1. Fraser, Lord, of Lonsdale. *My Story of St Dunstan's*, p.197.
2. Ibid, p.199.
3. Catran, Ken, and Penny Hansen. *Pioneering A Vision: A History of the Royal New Zealand Foundation for the Blind*, pp. 43–4.
4. Ibid.
5. From *Light in Darkness: A Brief History of the Jubilee Institute for the Blind: A Record of Great Achievements*. 1928. Auckland, New Zealand: Jubilee Institute for the Blind. Also from information supplied by Cyril Jenkin, early leader of The Commercial Travellers' and Warehousemen's Association of New Zealand, courtesy Theo V. Thomas, pp.279, 210, 211.
6. Fraser, op.cit., pp.280–82.
7. Ibid, p.208.
8. Ibid, p.210–11.

Chapter 21: Pearson and Helen Keller
1. Information supplied by Helen Keller International.
2. Keller, Helen Adams. *The Story of My Life*, p.10.
3. Ibid, p.30.
4. Ibid, p.41.
5. Ibid, p.57.
6. Helen Keller, speech at the Carnegie Hall, New York City, 5 January 1916.
7. Dark, Sidney. *The Life of Sir Arthur Pearson*, pp.196–200.

Chapter 22: Basil Gotto: In Memory of The Fallen
1. 'Basil Gotto', essay by Mark Quinlan, 2 December 2007.

Chapter 23: Richard King Huskinson
1. Richard King Huskinson. Obituary, *The New Beacon*, 15 May 1947, p.74.
2. King, Richard. *With Silent Friends*. London: John Lane, The Bodley Head.
3. Pearson, Sir Arthur. *Victory Over Blindness*, pp.307, 309–10, 314.
4. Shorter, Clement, in the Prefatory to Richard King's *With Silent Friends*.

Chapter 24: Death of the Chief
1. *The Times*, 12 December 1921.
2. Ibid, 10 December 1921.
3. Dark, Sidney. *The Life of Sir Arthur Pearson*, p.203.
4. *The Times*, 14 December 1921.
5. Ibid, 'Blindness as an Opportunity', 14 December 1921.
6. Dark, op.cit., pp.205–217.
7. Baden-Powell, Robert SS. 'The Late Sir Arthur Pearson', in *Headquarters Gazette*, January 1922.
8. Dark, op.cit., p.85.
9. Obituary, Cyril Arthur Pearson, *The Wykehamist*, 13 February 1922.

Chapter 25: Aftermath: Pearson's Legacy
1. *The Times*, 14 December 1921.
2. Fraser, Lord, of Lonsdale. *My Story of St Dunstan's*, p.313.

Epilogue
1. *New York Times*, 1 January 1922.
2. Sir Neville Pearson, 1958. Article written about his late father for the Scout Movement, in Heasman, pp.41-43.
3. *The Times*, 12 December 1921.
4. Ibid, 10 December 1921.
5. Pearson, Sir Arthur. *Victory Over Blindness*, viii.
6. Ibid, p.316.
7. Information supplied by Jean Norman (née Waldin.)
8. Goodchild, George (editor). *The Blinded Soldiers and Sailors Gift Book*.
9. The *Concise Oxford English Dictionary*.

Bibliography

Adams, James G. *Growing Up through the Great War*. Hull, UK: Bitterne Books, 2004

Baden-Powell, Robert SS. *Scouting for Boys*. Oxford: Oxford University Press, 2004

Berkeley, Reginald. *The History of the Rifle Brigade in the War of 1914–1918*. London: The Rifle Brigade Club Ltd, 1927

British Journal of Ophthalmology, Vol. 12, 1918.

Burns, Ross (editor). *The World War I Album*. London: Warfare, 1991

Castleton, D. *Blind Man's Vision*. London: St Dunstan's, 1990

Catran, Ken, and Penny Hansen. *Pioneering A Vision: A History of the Royal New Zealand Foundation for the Blind*. Auckland: RNZFB, 1992

Collins, Theresa M. *Otto Kahn*. Chapel Hill, NC, USA: University of North Carolina Press, 2002

Concise Oxford English Dictionary, London: BCA, 1996

Congreve, B. *Armageddon Road*. London: William Kimber, 1982

Cooper, Gladys. *Gladys Cooper*. London: Hutchinson and Co., 1931

Dark, Sidney. *The Life of Sir Arthur Pearson*. London: Hodder & Stoughton, 1922

Darwin, Charles. *The Origin of Species*. New York: Mentor Books, 1958

Everett, Percy W. *The First Ten Years*. Ipswich: The East Anglian Daily Times, 1948

Foli, Professor P. R. S. *Pearson's Dream Book*. London: C. Arthur Pearson Ltd, 1902

Foli, Professor P. R. S. *Pearson's Fortune-teller*. London: C. Arthur Pearson Ltd, 1902

Foli, Professor P. R. S. *Fortune Telling by Cards*. London: C. Arthur Pearson Ltd, 1902

Foli, Professor P. R. S. *Handwriting as an Index to Character*. London: C. Arthur Pearson Ltd, 1902

Fraser, Lord, of Lonsdale. *My Story of St Dunstan's*. London: George G. Harrap & Co. Ltd, 1961

Fraser, Lord, of Lonsdale. *Whereas I was Blind*. London: Hodder & Stoughton, 1942

Fry, C. B. *Life Worth Living*. London. Eyre & Spottiswoode, 1939

Gelder, Michael, Paul Harrison and Philip Cowen. *Shorter Oxford Textbook of Psychiatry*. Oxford University Press, 2006

Goodchild, George (editor). *The Blinded Soldiers and Sailors Gift Book*. London: Jarrold & Sons, 1921

Gotto, Basil. *Memoir* (unpublished).

Heasman, Robert. *Who was Cyril Arthur Pearson?* South Croydon, Surrey: Pearson's Holiday Fund, 2000

Herie, Euclid. *Journey to Independence*. Toronto: The Dundurn Group, 2005

Jubilee Institute for the Blind. *Light in Darkness: A Brief History of the Jubilee Institute for the Blind: A Record of Great Achievements*. Auckland, New Zealand: Jubilee Institute for the Blind, 1928

Keller, Helen Adams. *The Story of My Life*. New York: Doubleday, Page & Co., 1903

King, Richard. *With Silent Friends*. London: John Lane, The Bodley Head, 1917

Laffin, J. A. *A Western Front Companion*. Stroud, UK: Allan Sutton Publishing, 1994

Lawson, Sir Arnold. *War Blindness at St Dunstan's*. London: Henry Frowde, 1922

Menzies, Gavin. *1421: The Year China Discovered the World*. London: Bantam Press, 2002

McIlwain, J. *The Hospital of St Cross*. Andover, UK: Pitkin Pictorials, 1993

McIntosh, G. C. The Piri Reis Map of 1513. Athens, Georgia, USA: University of Georgia Press, 2000

Pearson, Sir Arthur. *Victory Over Blindness*. London: Hodder & Stoughton, 1919

Parker, Eric. *Hesketh Prichard*. London: T. Fisher Unwin, 1924

Prichard, Hesketh V. H. *Sniping in France*, London: Hutchinson & Co., 1922

Prichard, Hesketh V. H. *Through the Heart of Patagonia*. London: William Heinemann, 1902

Saint Dunstan's Annual. London: S.C.S., 5 Gower Street, 1935

St Dunstan's: A Story of Accomplishment.

Transactions of the American Ophthalmological Society, XVIII, 1920.

Upton, Chris. *Living Back-to-Back*. Trowbridge, UK: The Cromwell Press, 2005

Wallechinsky, D. *The Complete Book of the Olympics*. London: Aurum Press, 1996

War Diary of the 8th Rifle Brigade, The Royal Green Jackets' Museum, Winchester.

Watson, Frank L. (edited by C. B. Purdom). *Memoirs & Diaries: A Territorial in the Salient*. (First published in *Everyman at War*, edited by C. B Purdom. New York: Knopf Publishing Group, 1930)

Westlake, Roy. *Kitchener's Army*. Tunbridge Wells, UK: The Nutshell Publishing Co. Ltd, 1989

Winter, J. M. *The Experience of World War I*. London: Grange Books, 1988

Index

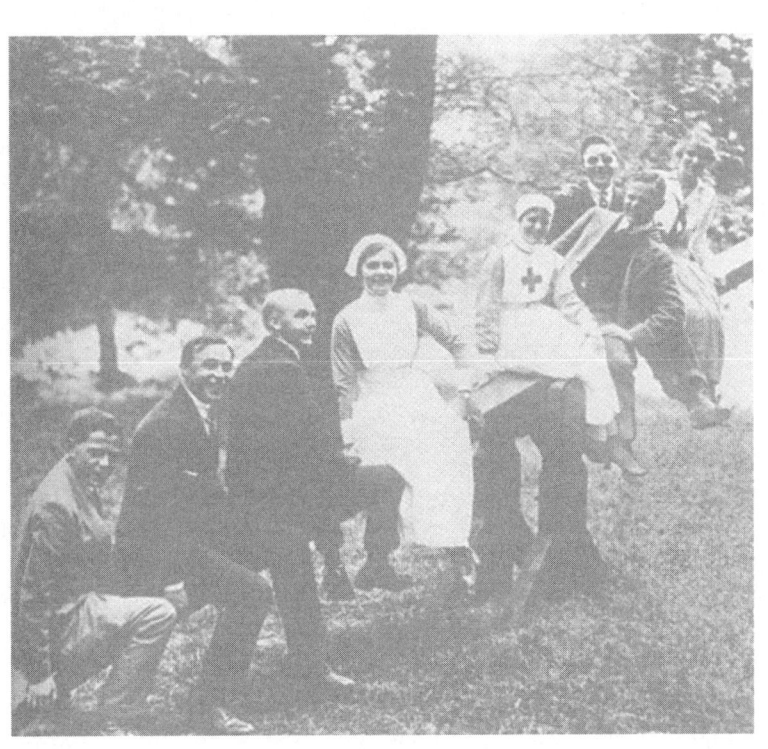